Managing Osteogenesis Imperfecta:

A Medical Manual

Edited by
Priscilla Wacaster, MD

Published by
The Osteogenesis Imperfecta Foundation, Inc.

ii

All correspondence and inquiries should be directed to:

Managing Osteogenesis Imperfecta: A Medical Manual
The Osteogenesis Imperfecta Foundation, Inc.
804 W. Diamond Avenue, Suite 210
Gaithersburg, MD 20878 USA

ISBN 0-9642189-3-3

52495 >

9 780964 218932

Funding for this project has been provided by the American Legion Child Welfare Foundation, Inc. In the 1950's, Dr. Garland D. Murphy, Jr., of Arkansas, worked with the American Legion's National Executive Committee to establish the Foundation. Dr. Murphy assigned to the Foundation deeds to fractional mineral rights on nearly 10,000 acres of land in the oil-rich Williston Basin in Montana and North Dakota.

The Foundation has two primary purposes – first, to contribute to the physical, mental, emotional, and spiritual welfare of children and youth through dissemination of knowledge about new and innovative organizations and/or their programs, and second, to make wider and more effective use of knowledge already possessed by well-established organizations, to the end that such information will benefit youth and be more adequately used by society.

The Osteogenesis Imperfecta Foundation, Inc., and its members thank Mr. Terry L. Woodburn and the American Legion Child Welfare Foundation, Inc., for their financial support of this book.

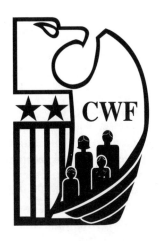

This book is dedicated to
my son, Neil, and to his
physical therapist,
Bev Housel, in gratitude
for her patience, kindness,
encouragement, and
friendship.

Preface
Preface
Preface
Preface
Preface

My goal as editor has been to provide something for everyone who treats patients with OI. The authors for each chapter have expertise in the particular field of medicine covered by that chapter. Most of them also have experience in caring for persons with OI. In addition, the main subject of each photograph in this book is a person with OI.

I would like to express my appreciation to the talented authors and to the many persons who have assisted me in typing, proofreading, and providing photographs for this text. I would also like to thank the American Legion Child Welfare

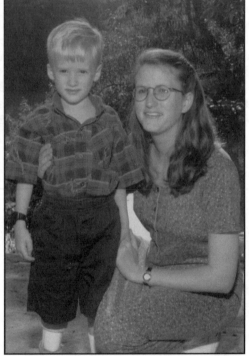

Photo by George Pongratz

Priscilla Ridgway Wacaster and son, Neil.

Foundation, Inc., for its financial support of this project and the Osteogenesis Imperfecta Foundation, Inc. and its wonderful staff for their unflagging support throughout the many months of this endeavor. Specifically, I want to thank Leanna Jackson for allowing me to be involved in this project and for all the many ways she helped me. Our typesetter, Judy Dodd, has been very patient and kind while teaching me the ins and outs of the publishing world. Thank you, Judy. I am eternally grateful to my husband, Jeff, and our son,

Neil, who have encouraged me and been tolerant of things (like having papers all over the house) while I was engrossed in this book.

Being a family physician has served me well in my role as editor. It provided the medical background needed to make this book one in which persons involved in different aspects of the medical care of children and adults with OI could find useful and informative facts. My greatest asset though is my intimate knowledge of the day to day management of persons with OI. My son and I both have Type I OI. I have been up all night with a two year old experiencing muscle spasms following a femur fracture. When he jumped for the first time ever as a four year old, I cheered – and then held my breath as he struggled to keep his balance! I have made countless trips to physicians, therapists, the pool, the radiology department at the hospital. As a young adult, I have suffered with arthritis. My hearing loss resulted in a stapedectomy in January, 1996. My son and I have personal experience with almost every topic addressed by this book. Therefore, I judged the manuscripts mostly in the light of how the information would be used to take care of people like us and our many friends who have OI.

It has been an honor for me to be involved in this project. I humbly offer this text to the OI community as a gift which I hope physicians and other caregivers will use to ease the burdens of families who live 24 hours a day with the realities of OI. May we have strength and compassion for the hard days and joy in each accomplishment.

Priscilla Ridgway Wacaster, MD

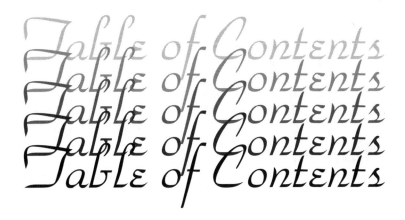

Table of Contents

x

Appendix A

Appendix B

Appendix C

Appendix D

Appendix E

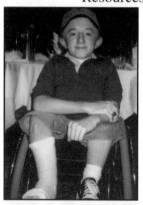

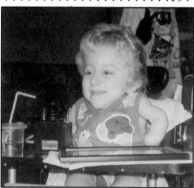

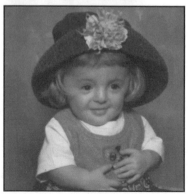

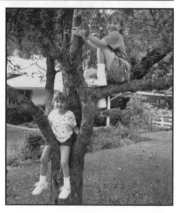

Chapter
Chapter
Chapter
Chapter
Chapter

1

Welcome to Osteogenesis Imperfecta

by Priscilla Wacaster, MD

Osteogenesis Imperfecta (OI) is a complex, dominantly inherited disorder of the collagen fiber itself or of the production of collagen. Joan Marini, MD, of the National Institutes of Health, refers to it as a medium rare disorder, the incidence in the general population being approximately 1:15,000 to 1:20,000 births.[1] A researcher from Australia, named D.O. Sillence, and his colleagues, have classified OI into four types: OI Type I is usually mild, with the person obtaining near normal to normal stature and frequently without severe deformity.[2] A person with OI Type II is frequently stillborn or dies prior to age one year, though some have survived to young adulthood. Multiple fractures and deformities are usually present at birth as well as an extremely soft cranium. OI Type III is often quite severe, with short stature, very fragile bones, and though some persons will achieve independent ambulation, most use wheelchairs, walkers, and/or braces for mobility. OI Type IV is considered to be somewhere in between Types I and III in severity. The terms "congenita" and "tarda" were used in the past but are no longer considered accurate.

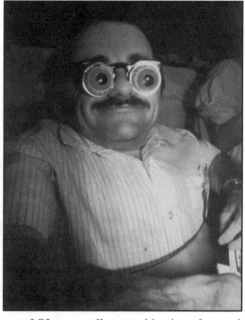

At the genetic level, the defect in the collagen synthesis may be a simple base pair substitution or a more complex error in an area of the gene which controls synthesis. OI Type I is usually a situation where the collagen fiber produced is normal but the quantity is quite low, therefore there is not enough collagen present for proper support of the connective tissue. The other types of OI are usually a combination of normal collagen produced by the normal allele for the gene and abnormally shaped collagen produced by the allele with the error.[1]

The gene is inherited in an autosomal dominant fashion. Some families have what appears to be recessive forms of the disorder. Recent research has indicated that mosaicism plays a role in some families where neither parent clinically appears affected, but more than one offspring is produced with clinically evident OI.[1,3]

This brief review of the genetics of OI is by no means exhaustive. The interested party is referred to one of the excellent genetic textbooks, such as Connective Tissue and Its Heritable Disorders, or to the myriad of medical literature on the subject for further technical information.

Now for a Review of Systems, or you may prefer to think of this as "Symptoms and Signs often seen in persons with OI."

Head – Often within normal limits of size for age, the head may appear relatively macrocephallic if the body is small for age. The face often has a triangular appearance. Hydrocephalus occurs in every person with Type II OI and a large percentage of persons with Type III OI.

Eyes – The blue sclerae may be quite prominent, or rather subtle, or completely absent. Evaluation by an ophthalmologist is advised as keratoconus, megalocornea, and corneal or lenticular opacities may occur. The person will probably be nearsighted. A ring similar to arcus senilis is often observed.

Ears – Conductive or sensorineural or mixed hearing loss is often seen prior to adulthood or in young adulthood – and is sometimes present by age three. Amplification or surgical intervention is often needed (see chapter 18). Surprisingly, children with OI may be very sensitive to loud sounds, especially music with a strong beat.

Nose – Frequent or spontaneous nose bleeds may occur.

Throat – Easy gag reflex which translates to difficulty swallowing pills is often seen. The person usually has a very high pitched voice. A rare complication is dentinogenesis imperfecta, which, if it occurs, will occur with the first tooth to erupt and will occur in each person in the family with OI. Therefore, it can be used as a diagnostic indicator in the families in which it occurs (see chapter 15). Temporomandibular joint (TMJ) disorders are sometimes present.

Back – Scoliosis can range from mild to severe enough to endanger breathing. Bracing is ineffective as the ribs usually bend rather than the vertebrae straightening. Internal fixation is sometimes warranted.

Chest – There may be respiratory compromise and/or decreased reserve secondary to barrel-chestedness. Rib fractures are common and can occur from a vigorous hug or a cough. Respiratory infection may lead to respiratory failure and death particularly in persons with OI Types II and III, therefore RSV bronchiolitis, bronchitis, or pneumonia is treated aggressively. Pectus excavatum may occur at birth with all types of OI and may spontaneously resolve within the first few months of life.

Cardiovascular – Murmurs may be due to ventricular septal defects at birth or may occur later in life due to mitral valve prolapse (see chapter 16). Aortic dissection has occurred in persons with OI.[4]

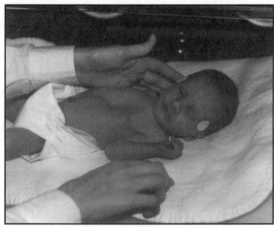

Newborn with Type I OI.

Skin – Often translucent with veins readily visible, the skin almost always bruises easily, and the person may sweat excessively and exhibit heat intolerance. Cartilage is quite pliable, and many caretakers find remarkable the softness of the skin. Sutures should be placed with the smallest possible subcuticular knots, needle size, and thread size, and external sutures should be removed as soon as possible. Some physicians have minimized scar width by using Steri-strips® across an area closed with subcuticular suturing. Pain tolerance, especially to bumps, scrapes, and bruises, may be very low.

Musculoskeletal – See chapters 2, 3, 5, 6 and 7. Often one is left to wonder, did the person fracture then fall or fall then fracture? The ease with which fractures can occur is startling especially if a fracture occurs while a caregiver is positioning the patient or removing a cast or even when operating on the patient. There have been witnessed fractures occurring in mid-air (non-weight bearing). Pre-teens are bothered by severe "growing pains" and all ages can have severe muscle cramps. Some people have had muscle cramps severe enough to cause a fracture. Flexeril® has been used successfully for relief of muscle cramps and spasms. Often one-half of a ten milligram tablet is sufficient as the person frequently has small body surface area. Muscle spasms can also be severe following fracture, particularly femur fracture. Benedryl® by mouth is quite effective in conjunction with adequate pain medicine for decreasing muscle spasms and promoting sleep, particularly in pre-schoolers. (The parents will thank you.) For pre-teens, Thorazine®, one-fourth of a ten milligram tablet orally, has been used effectively to relieve spasms and cramps. In the hospital, intramuscular Valium® is recommended for its ability to relieve the muscle spasms as well as decreasing the patient's anxiety and providing some amnesia for the frequently painful procedures the patient will have to endure (again, the family will thank you – even very young patients will have long memories of pain). Some persons with OI will have excessive callus formation following fracture, which can be quite dramatic. Most persons with OI will have hypermobile joints and can perform incredible feats, especially finger tricks. Persons should be counseled to perform these feats only in the presence of the physician, and caregivers should be aware of the hypermobility particularly when transferring the patient (ie. moving patient from bed to operating table).

Neurological – The baby is probably going to be very hypotonic with a Moro reflex which is very easy to elicit. As an older child or adult, the person may continue to startle easily, as well as being somewhat tremorous especially when under stress. A fine intention tremor can be seen especially if the person is nervous or excited. Intelligence is usually high normal to above normal, with many persons pursuing advanced degrees of study.

Genitourinary – Hypercalcuria is observed in some patients though

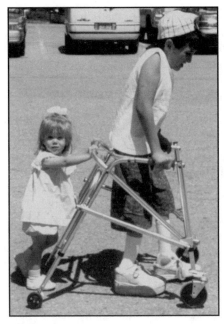

the clinical significance is not well delineated.[5] Renal calculi occasionally occur and should be suspected in a person with frequent urinary tract infections. **Gastrointestinal** – Constipation can be a problem at any age. A diet rich in fiber and fluids is highly recommended. Breastfeeding for as long as possible is also recommended as a deterrent to constipation, as well as the other usual benefits.

Endocrine – Some persons with OI will have low growth hormone levels. Some will respond to growth hormone therapy with increase in stature, and some will not (see chapter 13).

Anesthesia

Some people have the mistaken idea that since persons with OI fracture frequently that the fractures must not hurt as much. The adult or older child with a fracture may not be hysterical, but he or she is probably hurting. Younger children will often fall asleep if kept in a stable position only to awaken screaming when the fracture site is moved. Adequate pain medicine, whether acetaminophen with codeine by mouth or an injected narcotic, is necessary as soon as possible after presentation to the office or emergency room – even prior to x-ray. A few unfortunate persons with OI seem refractory to pain medicine and require what appear to be very high doses of narcotics to be able to refrain from screaming in pain.

The following are a few guidelines for anesthetic care. Premedication is vital especially for children.[6] While hospitalization and surgery is undoubtedly stressful for a child, it is also quite traumatic for the parents to have the child wheeled away, screaming in pain and distress. Versed® in its injectable liquid form can be given by mouth to children (0.25 to 0.75 mg/kg) prior to painful procedures such as skin biopsies and laceration repair, or as premedication for surgery.[7] Some persons with OI have a sensitivity to inhaled anesthetics such as halothane, which can cause hyperthermia.[6] Regional anesthesia is recommended though epidurals may suddenly become spinals secondary to the scoliosis.[6] Atropine can cause a drop in temperature and/or hyperventilation.

If one's operating room policies do not allow the parents in pre-op holding or the recovery room, consider changing the regulations or making a special exception for families dealing with OI. Ideally, a parent should be with the child until the child is asleep and when the child awakens. This usually results in a child who is calmer and more compliant with things such as oxygen masks and pulse oximeter clips.

Child Abuse

Child abuse, or non-accidental injury as it is currently termed in many circles, continues to be a problem in the United States. Many families with OI have been accused of child abuse, even to the children being removed from the home only to suffer more fractures while in protective custody. The decision to contact child protective services is difficult for a physician or other concerned person to make and is generally made with much forethought. The Osteogenesis Imperfecta Foundation is involved in an educational endeavor to encourage physicians evaluating a case which may include the possibility of child abuse to consider OI prior to calling social services. If there is no clinical evidence of OI, by all means, do what needs to be done to protect the child. But, if there is evidence of OI, for the family's and child's sake, investigate further, perhaps by calling in a geneticist or orthopaedist familiar with OI. It is much nicer to be remembered as "the physician who finally diagnosed our child," than as "the physician who falsely accused us of child abuse."

Paperwork (Everyone's Favorite Pastime!)

Organization is critical for the family with OI. Physicians and other caregivers can assist in this by offering copies of letters, clinic records, and test results. Encourage the families to keep all medical information together and to take their information with them whenever the affected person goes to see a physician. Relatively simple things, such as keeping a phone log of all conversations with the insurance company, can greatly increase the efficiency of the patient/insurance company relationship, especially if the patient is a member of an HMO. Many families carry a letter from their physician stating the existence of OI in an individual in order to avoid unpleasantness when treated in an unfamiliar emergency room.

Clinical Pearls or Advice From Somebody Who Figured This Out the Hard Way

1. Early intervention – If you do not know what it is and how to use it, read the article entitled "Pediatricians and early intervention: Everything

DECIDE FOR YOURSELF... IS THIS AN ABUSED CHILD?

A traumatized child

Unlikely or unsatisfactory explanation of how the fracture occurred

X-rays that reveal old fractures in various stages of healing

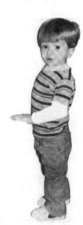

Evidence of Bruising

Varied types of fractures

Bones that appear normal on X-rays

NO, This child, like hundreds of children thought to have been abused, actually has Osteogenesis Imperfecta or Brittle Bone Disorder. At his current age of 10 he has experienced over 65 fractures. In distinguishing between child abuse and OI there are similarities, but please be aware of the important differences.*

- Blue Sclera, (whites of the eyes)
- Inverted triangular shaped skull
- Small stature
- Excessive mobility of the joints
- Thin fragile skin

- Excessive sweating
- Little soft tissue damage at fracture site
- Crush fractures of the vertebrae
- X-rays that reveal wormian bones
- Discolored, breakable teeth

*It is important to note that few patients with Osteogenesis Imperfecta (OI) show *all* of the listed abnormalities, and some show *none*. Some children with OI outwardly appear normal in every respect. A diagnostic test for OI in the form of a skin biopsy is available. It requires approximately 3 months to obtain results.

For more information, contact:
The Osteogenesis Imperfecta Foundation, Inc.
804 W. Diamond Avenue, Suite 210
Gaithersburg, MD 20878
(301) 947-0083

you need to know but are too busy to ask," by Richard Solomon, M.D. (*Infants and Young Children* 1995; 7(3):38-51).

2. Parents – You can trust them. Accept the parents, especially parents of a child with a disability, as colleagues. They are the primary care providers for their child as well as the persons who have specialized in the care of their child.

3. While most parents will prefer to do all of the handling of the child while in the office, the pediatrician or family physician caring for a child with OI should assign one nurse to perform all triage, injections, and other necessary interventions the child requires. One might even consider granting the nurse and family a few hours of the nurse's time, while on payroll, to interact with the child in the home. This will give the family more confidence when the child has to be handled at the office, and might result in a respite for the family if the nurse is willing to care for the child while the parents have an evening out (of course, the parents would pay the nurse then!).

4. Because of the complexity of treating persons with OI, you may need to instruct your staff to allow longer than average appointment times for your patients with OI.

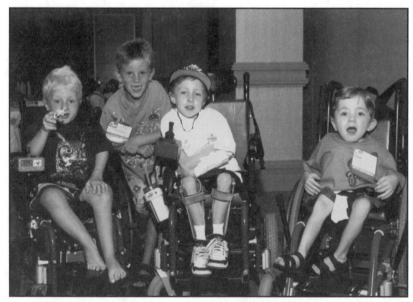

5. Ask yourself: If this were my child, would I do this without anesthesia or without Versed®/Valium® or without thorough explanation? Remember, you are not the last medical person this child will see. Make the experience as positive as possible. Your colleagues will appreciate it. Stated another way, treat the child as if you are the next medical person to walk in the room.

6. There is more to life than medical needs: Disabled parking stickers, child care (also termed respite care), financial concerns, social supports, etc. You may or may not be able to meet every need, but you can offer a listening ear and help the family get connected with someone who can address the need.

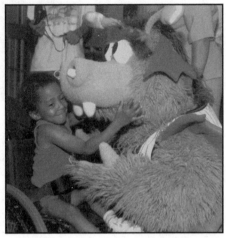

7. At first glance, the problems mentioned in the Review of Systems might seem overwhelming or depressing. Few individuals experience all of them in a lifetime yet often several are present at one time. In general, persons with OI live productive, self-supporting, fulfilling lives filled with friends and family. While one's life might be mildly or more severely affected by OI and its complications, I believe it to be a worthwhile existence.

8. A simple phone call or postcard sent after a fracture or surgery can go a long way in making you the best doctor in the world.

Recommendations for Check-ups

Vision by in office screening should be performed per usual routine with referral to ophthalmologist if visual irregularities occur.

Hearing should be evaluated by an audiologist experienced and trained in the evaluation of children at ages 3, 6, and 10, then by an audiologist every 2 years until 20 years of age, then yearly.

Developmental assessment should be performed at every well baby check with referral to early intervention providers at the first hint of a delay.

Immunizations and well child checks should be as per routine.

Scoliosis checks should begin in preschool years for persons with OI Types II, III, and IV and in pre-teen years for persons with OI Type I.

Dental examination should be performed by a qualified dentist at the eruption of the first tooth or by age one, whichever comes first.

The usual routine of Pap smears should be followed, as should one's typical recommendations for contraception including counseling for male and female teenagers and young adults. There is no contraindication to the pelvic examination of a woman with OI, though prudence, such as the use of gentle technique and an appropriately sized speculum, is recommended.

There are no specific laboratory discrepancies known to be associated with OI though some persons will have platelet dysfunction, alkaline phosphatase elevation, or hypercalcuria. Screening laboratory studies should be performed as per routine.

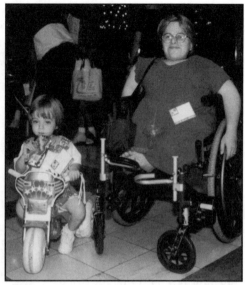

This woman and her daughter both have OI.

References

[1] Marini J, MD. "The First Osteogenesis Imperfecta Support Group," MCV Pediatric Grand Rounds, Richmond, Virginia, February 13, 1996.

[2] Sillence DO, Senn A, Danks DM. Genetic heterogeneity in osteogenesis imperfecta. J Med Genet, 1979;16:101-116.

[3] Byers PH., Wallis GA, Willing MC. Osteogenesis imperfecta: Translation of mutation to phenotype. J Med Genet, 1991;28:433-442.

[4] Moriyama Y., et. al. Acute aortic dissection in a patient with osteogenesis imperfecta. Ann Thorac Surg, 1995;60:1397-1399.

[5] Vetter U, et. al. Osteogenesis imperfecta in childhood: Cardiac and renal manifestations. Eur J Pediatr, 1989;149:184-187.

[6] Masuda Y, et. al. Anesthetic management of a patient with osteogenesis imperfecta congenita. Masui, 1990;39:383-387. (Abstract in English, manuscript in Japanese)

[7] Feld LH, et. at. Oral midazolam preanesthetic medication in pediatric outpatients. Anesth, 1990;73:831-834.

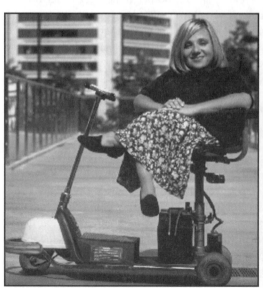

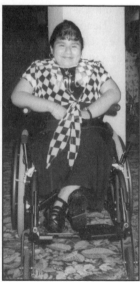

Chapter
Chapter
Chapter
Chapter
Chapter

2

Bone
Basics

by Paul Sponseller, MD

I. Introduction

Bone is an important tissue in the human body. If it could be given a personality, one would say it is the strong, silent type. It never makes its presence felt unless there is a problem. Bone provides form. The overall height and shape of the body is determined primarily by the length and shape of the underlying skeleton. In addition, bone provides stability to the body. It provides the strength for standing, as well as a fulcrum for muscles to act upon, transmitting power. When muscles generate movements in various parts of the body, they act on the bones which then move in a coherent pattern. Bone is not present from the start during the development of the human. In the embryo, the skeleton is a smaller version of itself, almost completely formed in cartilage. The head is relatively large at this stage and grows somewhat in the future, whereas the trunk and limbs are relatively small but catch up during later growth. The cartilage gradually calcifies in a pattern, first in the center (the diaphysis of the bones) then at the ends of the bones (the epiphyses). All that is left of this cartilage in a child, is the smooth cartilage on the joint surfaces, as well as the cartilage growth plates near either end which allow increase in length throughout growth. Finally, in adulthood, even these cartilage remnants are gone: the growth plate closes and turns to bone at the end of puberty, and the cartilage on joint surfaces usually starts to wear out in later life through continued use. Bone, by contrast, is the only tissue which can heal and repair itself with identical structure. When a bone breaks, it heals and forms new bone. Bone eventually remodels to match the original bone. Similarly, when a bone is cut during surgery, the same process happens. No other tissue in the body heals quite this same way. This is because bone is an active tissue.

In the body, bone bears little resemblance to the dry brittle bone one sees in a skeleton. Bone is living. It is filled with cells and has a tremendous blood supply to support its growth and function. Bone is continuously being remodeled to meet the stresses placed upon it. Some cells within the bone (osteoblasts) form new bone when more strength is needed or when a repair process is necessary. By contrast, other cells, osteoclasts, remove bone when it is not necessary. This happens when one changes from an active to sedentary life-style. It also happens after approximately age 35, as the aging process causes us to lose some of our bone density. Being more active results in more bone strength; being less active makes the bone more brittle. In addition, building blocks such as calcium, phosphorus, and vitamin D and signals such as hormones, affect how strong the bones are. However, most bone disorders seen today are not a result of deficiencies in these areas and therefore adding more building blocks or calcium, phosphorus, and vitamin D does not help to strengthen the bone if the primary problem is not a deficiency.

Bone has a shape which is familiar to all, from pictures of skeletons. There is a thick outer layer called the cortex which is especially thick in the middle of long weightbearing bones such as the femur or tibia. In addition, it has a spongy center, filled with a lattice work of bone called the medullary canal. At the ends of the bone are the epiphyses. These are covered with smooth joint cartilage to produce the gliding motion of joints. The bones are held together with ligaments which attach directly and allow motion but prevent dislocation. Looking at bone under the microscope is very hard because the bone is difficult to section unless the calcium is dissolved out. This can be done using hydrochloric acid. This results in a more spongy connective tissue foundation. The majority of the noncalcified portion of

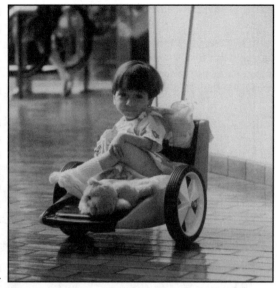

bone is made out of collagen. Collagen is a strand-like connective tissue which is used to build the shape or structure of bone and is later calcified. Collagen is made out of three polypeptides, each with over a thousand amino acids. These fibrils are quite small and laid together in overlapping strands. At the junctions of the overlapping strands, the calcium and phosphorus are deposited.

The three polypeptides form a spiral shape. This is called a triple helix. The majority of collagen in bone is called type I collagen. Procollagen is formed in the cells and extruded out into the surrounding matrix where it can perform its function of building the bone. After it is extruded from the cell, it undergoes several biochemical changes or modifications. It is changed from procollagen to collagen. It changes from aggregated random alignment to a straight strand-like structure. It is the collagen, which is missing one or more critical amino acids, which is abnormal in Osteogenesis Imperfecta (OI). As discussed in other chapters, the specific type of defect varies from patient to patient.

II. Bone in Osteogenesis Imperfecta

In Osteogenesis Imperfecta, the bone is more slender (gracile) than in other people. The cortex is thin and is not as strong. There is a cortical layer but often it is porous. There is relative osteoporosis. The epiphysis is essentially normal and the growth plate is normal. However, there are clumps of calcified cartilage inside the end of the growth plate. The vertebrae of the spine are often quite flattened due to the large amount of stress placed during daily sitting and bearing weight. Fortunately, the discs are preserved and there is no significant chance of a slipped disc in an OI patient. The flattened vertebrae are one of the causes of short stature of the trunk. The blood supply of the bone in Osteogenesis Imperfecta is abundant. This may cause it to bleed more during surgery than in average bone.

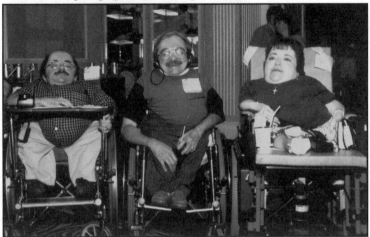

The bone will often develop microfractures as the patient puts weight upon it. A microfracture is a partial crack to the bone which may not produce much, if any pain and no observable severe deformities. However, multiple microfractures over time can gradually lead to an increased bowing of the bone which may finally fracture. This often occurs in patients with Osteogenesis Imperfecta and is a cause of bowing of the legs and sometimes the arms. The frequency of fractures increases as the child becomes more active but eventually decreases in most patients during adulthood. Fractures may still occur throughout life but the frequency is decreased after maturity.

Also in Osteogenesis Imperfecta, it is important to realize that collagen is present in the ligaments. This is the reason the ligamentous laxity occurs and gives rise to scoliosis (a spinal curvature) in a large number of patients. It can also cause instability or giving out of the knee or other joints.

If one takes a sample of Osteogenesis Imperfecta bone to look under the microscope, there are some abnormalities. The bone thickness is more slender and the bone trabeculae do not always connect together, but are more random. There is more woven bone indicating frequent fractures and remodeling.

Once a fracture occurs in a patient with Osteogenesis Imperfecta, it normally heals in a standard period of time. The bone is just as strong after it heals, as it was before. The only exception to that is if there is a lot of bowing in the bone, then even the normal stresses in the bone are likely to predispose it to refracture.

The types of fractures seen in a patient with Osteogenesis Imperfecta are not much different than people with normal collagen. Patients with Osteogenesis Imperfecta can have a spiral fracture or a buckle fracture or a straight (transverse) fracture. Therefore, there is no type of fracture specific to Osteogenesis Imperfecta.

Bone biopsy can sometimes be used to prove the diagnosis of Osteogenesis Imperfecta but there are many OI patients where an abnormality still cannot be found because the scientific techniques are not fully developed. Therefore, bone biopsies do not have a normal role in the care of the individual patient with OI. Its role is more in research and understanding of OI.

When an orthopaedic surgeon first sees a patient who may have OI, (s)he must first think of other conditions which can mimic it. The first is rickets. Rickets is decreased calcification and development of the bone due to a diet deficient in vitamin D, or due to its handling of these components in the body. Another cause to consider is hyperpituitarism. This is a rare disorder in which an excessive pituitary hormone can cause dissolving of the bone. Finally, Mendes' Syndrome can cause similar changes in the bone.

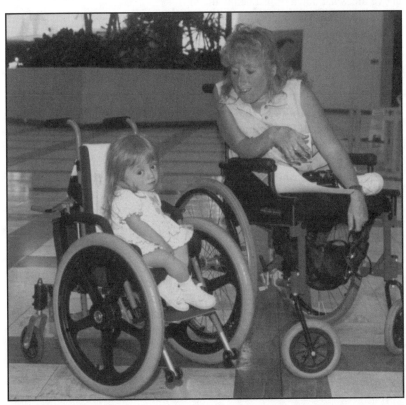

III. Treatment

The treatment for Osteogenesis Imperfecta is still being researched. Currently, there is no technique which can reverse the basic defect in the collagen and make it normal. Current treatments involve supporting the bone to make it more functional. In other chapters, you will read about insertion of rods. It is important to have a normal diet including calcium, phosphorous, and vitamin D. However, adding these in excessive quantities will not help the bone. Previous trials have included vitamin D and calcitonin (hormone) injections. They did not show any noticeable difference and are therefore not currently used in the management of patients with OI. However, there are many new developments on the horizon. Some of these developments resemble those used in patients with osteoporosis, as seen in the elderly. It is quite likely that more effective therapy will be developed to strengthen the bone of patients with OI.

Supportive treatment includes bracing for standing, in children who have weaknesses of the muscles and significant bowing of the bones. Standing can help build the bone up to a limited extent. Bracing may be from above the waist down or just below the hips.

Electrical stimulation of bone has not been shown to make bone stronger in persons with Osteogenesis Imperfecta. However, in some cases it can help heal a fracture which is slow to heal or has stopped healing.

A very important part of treatment is to have a good physical therapist for children who are late in learning to walk. The therapist can help improve strength, improve standing balance, give reassurance, and monitor for fractures and deformities. They can help to assist with the use of braces. Each person should have an individualized plan for how much need there is for physical therapy.

Understanding and treating persons with OI is a team approach. The family, therapist, orthopaedist, and generalist all work together. We are heartened to observe that many people with OI lead productive, accomplished lives.

Chapter Chapter Chapter Chapter Chapter 3

Imaging in Osteogenesis Imperfecta

by M. Ines Boechat, MD

How Much Radiation Is Safe?

Patients and their parents frequently ask how much radiation is safe, how much is too much, and what can be done to control the amount used. Is there a number which, when exceeded, causes danger to life or future generations? There are no easy answers. All persons are exposed to measurable amounts of radiation in their environment. Sources include cosmic radiation, natural terrestrial radiation, and radiation emanating from chemical elements within the body. There is considerable variation within North America and among various geographic locations around the world with respect to the measurable amounts of natural background radiation; background radiation levels vary severalfold within the continental United States, and higher levels are found in other countries. Exposure to these amounts of low-level environmental background radiation is unavoidable.

Many in the lay community are of the opinion that any amount of radiation exposure has adverse biologic effects, and therefore that reductions in exposure to even the lowest level of background radiation reduces the risk of adverse effects. There are no objective data, however, to support this view. Information pertaining to cancer rates in subjects living in geographic regions with differing levels of background radiation does not support the contention that variations in the level of background radiation are related to differences in cancer rates among human populations. Thus, subjects living in areas where levels of background radiation are relatively low do not have reduced rates of malignancy. Conversely, there is no increase in the frequency of cancer in populations residing in areas with relatively higher levels of background radiation.[1]

Medical radiation accounts for approximately 15% of the annual radiation exposure in the United States, including radiation therapy and nuclear medicine. The amount of additional radiation exposure provided by radiographic diagnostic procedures must be evaluated within the context of radiation exposure from all sources, including background radiation. Statements about doses of radiation associated with various x-ray procedures lose meaning without a quantitative frame of reference. It is very difficult to give an exact measurement of the true radiation to a given person without knowing all the details of that person's size and the type of study performed. This is why there is no simple answer to the question often asked regarding the radiation dose a child will receive from a specific examination.

The unit of radiation used to refer to x-ray exposures is the millirem, which is one thousandth of a rem. Rads and rems are units of absorbed dose of radiation. The rem includes a factor which relates specifically to the effect of the radiation on the human body. Rad stands for radiation absorbed dose and rem stands for radiation equivalent in man. For diagnostic x-rays, one rad equals one rem. These terms are still used to express radiation dosages, although new international units called Grays and Sieverts are now being adopted. One Gray is equivalent to 100 rads, and one Sievert is 100 rems.

Table 1 provides examples of radiation doses for chest and spine x-rays for children at different ages, and compares them with the natural background radiation and the exposure to cosmic radiation during a transcontinental flight.[2]

Table 1

Whole body equivalent doses or millirems (mrem) for children at different ages.

Exam	Age (years)		
	5	**10**	**20**
Chest x-ray	4.4	3.9	3.2
Lumbar Spine			
Anteroposterior	2.1	2.0	1.8
Lateral	13.1	12.1	11.2
Natural background			
per month	22.4	18.1	10.7
Transcontinental flight	3.7	3.0	1.8

The physician requesting an examination weighs the risk of radiation exposure to the benefit obtained by the information provided by the x-ray study. Radiographs are commonly used to assist in the early diagnosis of many diseases and injuries; they are extensively used in the evaluation of patients with Osteogenesis Imperfecta (OI). The radiographic changes that are used to classify patients with OI, such as progressive scoliosis, develop over the years and there is a marked variation in these changes.[3] It is not possible to predict at birth the final type of disease that will develop in any patient, therefore the patient has to be examined many times. Moreover, patients with OI are at risk for multiple fractures, development of bone deformities, and scoliosis, which are diagnosed and followed with x-rays.

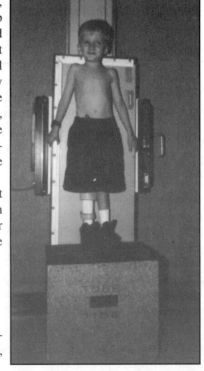

Responsible parents do their best to minimize the risk of radiation exposure to themselves and their children and some precautions can be suggested.

Preparing Children for Imaging Studies

The most common x-ray examinations, such as of the chest or bones, require little or no advance preparation. Children may be frightened by the examination room surroundings and parental reassurance with simple explanations about the "picture" to be taken usually suffice. Parents should always stress how important it is for the child to hold very still, while the x-ray is being taken, so that the image will be sharp and clear and the study does not have to be repeated.

Immobilization devices are frequently used to obtain correct positioning of children and decrease the number of repeat exposures. Parents should advise technologists of their child's condition, so that careful manipulation avoids further trauma. The technologist may recruit the parent's assistance in order to position a very fragile child. Children can often tell where it hurts, and the technologist's attention is then focused to the area so that the radiograph accurately depicts a new fracture.

Gonadal shielding should be considered anytime that the gonads are within the primary beam of radiation. Gonadal protection is achieved in a most effective way by tight collimation of the x-ray beam at the time of examination, but actual covering of the gonads with leaded devices is also a recommended practice. The use of shields, however, may obscure important anatomic details. In boys, the testes can be shielded in almost all examinations of the abdomen and pelvis; in girls, however, shielding is not practical in most examinations, since the ovaries are near other structures that need to be evaluated, such as pelvic bones and sacrum. Parents should consult the technologist performing an examination about the feasibility of gonadal shielding before each study.[4] When staying within a one foot area from the x-ray beam, parents should wear lead aprons to protect against scattered radiation, which may be present in very small doses.

What Are the Most Common Indications for X-ray Examinations in Patients With OI?

1. Skeletal Survey

The complete skeletal survey is most useful for evaluating patients with OI. Images of the entire body are obtained when the diagnosis is first suspected and should include views of the skull, spine, pelvis, and extremities in the anteroposterior (AP) projection, plus additional lateral views of the skull and spine. Although some of the views can be combined in small infants, a single view of the entire baby is not recommended, since positioning and examination quality in such cases is poor.[5] Standard doses are used and should not be modified because the child is osteopenic, allowing the appreciation of changes in density over time by the radiologist.

2. Fractures

Children with OI have fragile bones that can easily fracture. X-rays are essential in the evaluation of a fracture, indicating its exact location, if more than one bone is involved and if there is displacement of the fragments. During the healing process, the x-rays will show the presence of a bony callus, which indicates repair of the fracture, if the alignment of the bones is correct, and if deformities have developed.

3. Scanogram

This is a special type of x-ray, which is used to measure the actual size of the extremities. Patients with OI may develop bowing of the long bones as part of the disease process, or secondary to a fracture. Measurement of the leg length discrepancy is necessary for treatment planning. A very long film is used in a special film cassette measuring 14 x 36 inches. A ruler with radiopaque centimeter marker is placed on the cassette surface and the child lays upon it with the extremities securely immobilized and as flat as possible. An x-ray is then taken, producing an image of both the bones and the ruler. Therefore, accurate measurements of both extremities can be performed and the referring physician is given the information about the difference in length between the right and left legs.

Another method to obtain the same results is through a computed tomography (CT scan) examination. The child lays on the CT scan table and a computerized x-ray image is taken. With the help of electronic calipers, the technologist does the same measurements of the right and left extremity and the computer provides the total difference in length. The amount of radiation exposure is less than half of the dose delivered by the traditional x-ray method, and the study can be performed in approximately 15 minutes.[6]

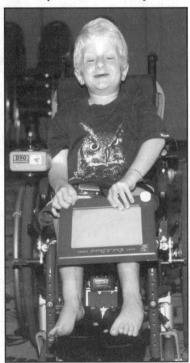

4. Scoliosis Films

Children with OI frequently develop scoliosis, an abnormal debilitating curvature of the spine. Patients with scoliosis undergo between two to six examinations during their evaluation and treatment. In many Radiology Departments around the country, 14 x 17 or 14 x 36 inches films are used for evaluation of the spine, and the cassette employed to hold these films is placed in a track built into the wall of the examining room, allowing height adjustments several different ways: anteroposterior (AP), lateral, and with flexion/extension. The use of this very long film allows appreciation of the degree of curvature of the spine on the AP projection, as well as the alignment of the head and shoulders in relation to the pelvis. This standing view allows evaluation of pelvic tilt and the influence of leg length discrepancy. Upright views are more important than views with the child laying down, because the degree of curvature increases with weight bearing. The lateral view should also be carefully examined for the presence of kyphosis ("hunchback"), which is frequently associated with scoliosis and may go unnoticed from the frontal view alone. The angle of curvature or scoliosis, is then measured according to one of several methods available and treatment decisions are made. Another function of these films is to evaluate the presence of anatomic abnormalities.

A new technology, using stimulable phosphor imaging plates (Computed Radiograph or CR) instead of the ordinary film-screen combination, allows significant reduction of the radiation dose in scoliosis examinations, while providing good visualization of the anatomic structures. This method has also possible benefits of radiation exposure reduction up to 40% of the original dose and a lower repeat dose, because the digital images can be adjusted by the computer before printing. As more centers in 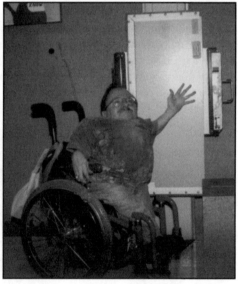 the country adopt this technique, more patients will benefit from these advantages.[7,8]

5. Computerized Tomography (CT) and Magnetic Resonance Imaging (MRI)

These methods provide cross-sectional images of the body; CT uses a thin beam of x-rays detected by a computer, while MRI is based on a combination of magnetic fields and radiowave signals also detected and integrated by a computer. CT and MRI are indicated in the evaluation of patients with OI when they develop neurological signs. Basilar impression of the soft occipital bone may cause hydrocephalus or brain stem pressure with foramen magnum compression.

6. Nuclear Medicine Studies

An isotope scan, also known as a nuclear scan, is usually performed in the nuclear medicine department of a hospital. A very small dose of a radioactive isotope, specific for a particular organ, is injected into a vein. It accumulates in the target organ and, after a preset time, the patient is placed under a radiation detector called a gamma camera, which records the radiation coming from the patient. The radioactive material used for the procedure gradually loses its activity over time and does not represent a risk to the patient.

These studies are not commonly requested for patients with OI. Sometimes, the doctors may suspect the presence of a bone infection, and a bone scan will be performed. Or a bone scan may be requested to depict the whole skeleton and areas of increased uptake of radioisotope, indicative of new fractures.

Conclusion

There are many imaging modalities for the evaluation of patients with Osteogenesis Imperfecta. The radiologist is a consultant to the primary physician on how to select the best examination for the specific problem presented, and a parent's ally for the well-being of their child.

References

[1] Gilsanz V, Roe TF, Goodman W. Does radiation research in healthy children pose greater than minimal risk? IRB 1994;16(5):6-8.

[2] Cann CE. Why, when and how to measure bone mass: A guide for the beginning user. In: Expanding the Role of Medical Physics in Nuclear Medicine, Frey GD, Yester MV, (eds.) Washington, D.C., American Physics Institute, 1991:250-279.

[3] Hanscon DA, et. al. Osteogenesis imperfecta: Radiographic classification, natural history and treatment of spinal deformities. J Bone Joint Surg 1992;74:598-616.

[4] O'Connell AM, Leone NM. Your child and x-rays: A parent's guide to radiation, x-rays, and other imaging procedures. Lion Press 1988:15-22.

[5] Poznanski AK. Practical approaches to pediatric radiology. Year Book Medical Publishers 1976:(P)313.

[6] Huurman WW, Jacobsen FS, Anderson JC, et. al. Limb-length discrepancy measured with computerized axial tomographic equipment. J Bone Joint Surg 1987;69A:699-705.

[7] Jonsson A, Jonsson K, Eklund K, et. al. Computed radiography in scoliosis: Diagnostic information and radiation dose. Acta Radiol 1995;36:429-433.

[8] Stringer DA, Calms RA, Poskitt KJ, et. al. Comparison of stimulable phosphor technology and convention screen-film technology in pediatric scoliosis. Pediatr Radiol 1994;24:1-5.

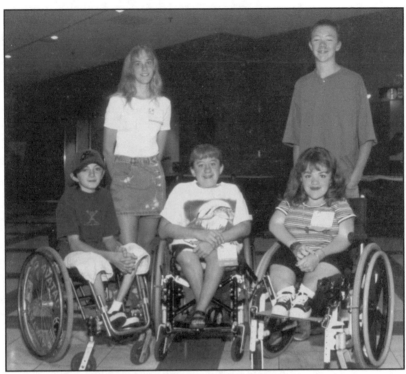

Group of teenagers at OI Convention in Orlando, Florida.
Note the difference in muscle mass of the teens.

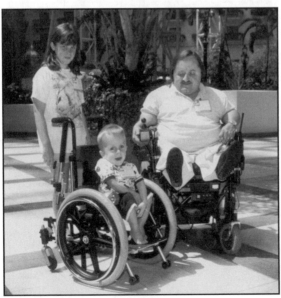

Conference attendees in Orlando, Florida.

Chapter

4

Quantitative Radiology

by Thomas N. Hangartner, PhD

The quantitative radiological methods for the assessment of bones are based on carefully recorded images obtained with x-rays. The expectation is that radiologically evaluated bone density is directly related to bone strength and can indicate the probability of fractures. We will first describe the various clinically available methods and explain what information can be obtained from these images. We will then review these imaging characteristics in relationship to Osteogenesis Imperfecta (OI) and assess their usefulness in diagnosing OI and quantifying the degree of brittleness of bone.

Radiologic Methods

Plain film radiographs have been used for many decades to assess fractures and their healing. A loss of bone density, however, can only be observed with the naked eye if it amounts to at least 30%.[1] For this reason, more sophisticated methods are needed to assess bone density.

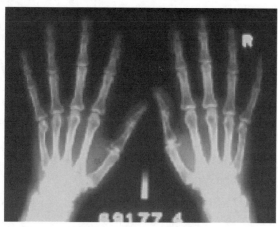

Fig. 1 Hand radiograph with aluminum wedge positioned between the hands. This type of image is the basis for radiographic absorptiometry.

The concurrent exposure of an aluminum wedge when taking a radiograph of the hands (Fig. 1) allows a normalization of the gray values of the film to equivalent aluminum thickness. This method, known as *radiographic absorptiometry* (RA), analyzes the phalanges.[2] The result represents the amount of bone in a chosen cross-section (Fig. 2).

Possible inhomogeneities in film exposure and development can introduce errors in the gray level calibration. *Single photon absorptiometry* (SPA) circumvents this problem by using a photon detector in place of a film.[3] A focused beam of x-ray photons scans parts of the forearm in a rectilinear pattern (Fig. 3). In order to avoid the influence of soft tissue overlying the bone, the forearm is put in a water bath or wrapped

Fig. 2 Cross-sectional view of a finger bone being imaged on an x-ray film as used in radiographic absorptiometry. The projection represents at each point the summed density values encountered by the x-ray beam along its path to the film. The bone mineral content is proportional to the area under the projection curve after subtraction of the soft-tissue area.

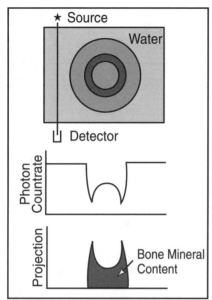

Fig. 3 Schematic illustration of a bone measurement by single-photon absorptiometry. Only the bone material contributes to a change in the measured photon count rate. The count-rate profile can be mathematically transformed into a projection profile of bone density. The area under this curve represents the bone mineral content.

into a soft-tissue equivalent, gelatinous material. Again, the obtained result represents the amount of bone in a cross-section whose location is defined by the position of a given scan line.

In order to avoid the water bath and make other bones such as spine or femur accessible for measurements, *dual-energy absorptiometry* methods have been developed. Depending on the type of radiation source used, they are known as dual-photon absorptiometry (DPA)[4] or dual energy x-ray absorptiometry (DXA or DEXA).[5] A scanning process generates the images that can be evaluated in a similar way as those of the previously discussed methods (Fig. 4). It has become customary to extract two parameters that are closely related to each other. The first is bone mineral content (BMC), giving the amount of bone present in an individual vertebra or in a specified region of interest in the femur or other bones. It is possible to scan the whole body and calculate the total weight of one's bones. The second parameter divides the BMC value by the area of the region of interest and expresses this as bone mineral density (BMD). The unit for BMD is g/cm^2, i.e., mass of bone per projected area (Fig.5).

Both BMC and BMD are dependent on the size of the bones which are usually related to the size of the patient. This dependence applies to all bone measurement methods discussed so far.

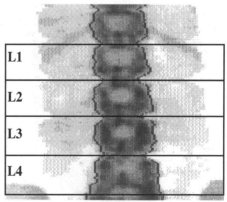

Fig. 4 Sample image of a spine measured by dual-energy absorptiometry. Of the five vertebrae shown, only L-1 to L-4 are usually evaluated for clinical purposes.

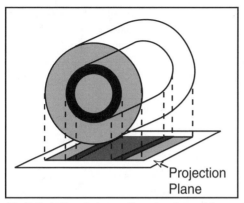

Fig. 5 Projection of a bone with surrounding soft tissue onto a plane. If created with a dual-energy scanner, the soft tissue layer can be accurately subtracted, providing a projected image of just the bone.

A patient of small stature and normal bones will produce the same measured values as a patient of large stature but low-density bones. It is, therefore, customary to take body size into account when interpreting the results of these measurements. The body size correction, however, is based on an average relationship of bone size to body size, and there can be considerable differences between a certain individual and the average population.

A body-size independent measurement of bone density is the assessment of the amount of bone per volume element, expressed in g/cm³. This assessment can be done by measuring cross-sectional images with a *computed tomography* (CT) scanner. Because the images are evaluated quantitatively, these methods are known as QCT. For the assessment of the vertebrae, a whole-body CT scanner is used.[6] A phantom containing bone- and soft-tissue-like material is scanned concurrently with the patient and used for calibration of the resulting values. Smaller CT scanners[7] are employed for the measurement of peripheral bones (pQCT), i.e., arms and legs (Fig.6).

The major advantage of bone density measurements by CT is the ability to separate cortical and trabecular bone. This is possible because CT provides a three-dimensional representation of the bone if several adjacent slices are measured. Even for a single slice, the image gives the correct representation of the measured cross-section (Fig. 7). This is in contrast to all other methods described which give a two-dimensional projection of the three-dimensional structure. In the two-dimensional projection, cortical and trabecular bone are overlying each other and cannot be separated.

Imaging Characteristics and OI

The weakening of bones affected by OI is primarily based on a defect in the collagen matrix. How this defect influences bone mineralization and bone size is presently not clear. The strength of a bone depends both on the strength of the bone material and the architecture of the bone. The architecture, including bone size, thickness of cortex as well as relative abundance of trabeculae and their thickness, is difficult to assess separately from the material density of bone if one uses projection methods. Only CT can separate these two components. It might be possible, however, to obtain a good indicator for bone strength with projection methods if the measured combination of density and architecture reflects the overall weight-bearing capacity of the bone. There is a need for more research to prove this relationship before the results of projection methods can be used as indicators for bone strength in OI.

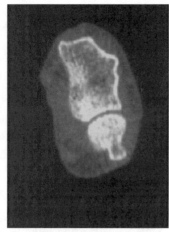

Fig. 6 Cross-sectional image of a forearm, measured close to the distal end by a pQCT scanner. Radius (larger bone) and ulna are shown.

Some recent studies using DEXA show that children with mild OI, as a group, have reduced bone mass values in the spine compared with controls.[8,9] However, body weight is an important factor to be considered, and the separation between the two groups is too small to provide a high reliability of identifying OI on an individual basis. Another study using SPA came to the conclusion that bone mass measurements in the forearm are not indicative for OI in the mild form of the disease.[10]

The ability of computed tomography to assess architecture is based on the fact that thin slices are imaged through the bone. These slices have generally a geometric resolution that allows accurate assessment of bone size, cortical thickness, average trabecular density, and cortical material density. Only special scanners can assess the trabecular architecture. However, with the reasonable assumption that the material density of trabecular bone is the same as that of cortical bone, it is possible to calculate what percentage of the trabecular region is actually covered by bone material.

The material density of bone needs to be assessed in the cortex, where the limited geometric resolution does not adversely affect the results. Special analysis procedures are necessary which have been proven to work on whole-body and peripheral CT scanners.[11] Children with OI have shown drastically reduced values in cortical material density.[12] In these patients, the trabecular density was also low, but there were a number of subjects

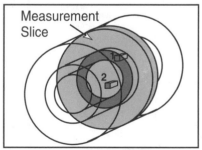

Fig. 7 Illustration of a thin slice as measured by CT. Individual elements can be attributed either to cortical (1) or trabecular (2) bone, allowing a separate evaluation of these two bone compartments.

without OI who had equally low trabecular bone density. There are indications that, in the mild form of OI, the cortical material density increases with age without concurrent increase of the trabecular density.[13] This shows that it will be helpful to analyze cortical and trabecular bone separately. The only method currently available that can achieve this is CT.

Conclusion

The quantitative radiologic assessment of bone in OI is still considered to be experimental. Whereas low resulting values are often interpreted as a reduction in strength, it is conceivable to obtain normal radiologic values from a patient with OI with reduced bone strength. There is great need for additional research that combines mechanical testing with radiographic assessment and computer modeling of bone samples that vary in material properties and architecture.

Editor's Note: The analysis of images obtained by whole-body and peripheral CT scanners as discussed above are presently only available at Dr. Hangartner's laboratory in Ohio. Despite problems associated with being body size dependent, dual energy x-ray absorptiometry (DEXA) is the most commonly used method for the determination of bone density in children and adults and is available at most major medical centers in the United States.

References
[1] Lachman E. Osteoporosis: The potentialities and limitations of its roentgenologic diagnosis. Am J Roentgenol 1955;74:712-715.
[2] Colbert C, Bachtell RS. Radiographic absorptiometry (photodensitometry). Cohn, SH. Noninvasive measurements of bone mass and their clinical application. Boca Raton, Florida, CRC Press, Inc. 1981:51-84.
[3] Cameron JR, Sorenson J. Measurement of bone mineral in vivo: an improved method. Science 1963;142:230-232.
[4] Peppler WW, Mazess RB. Total body bone mineral and lean body mass by dual photon absorptiometry. I. Theory and measurement procedure. Calcif Tissue Int 1981;33:353-359.
[5] Mazess RB, Collick B, Trempe J, et al. Performance evaluation of a dualenergy x-ray bone densitometer. Calcif Tissue Int 1989;44:228-232.
[6] Cann CE, Genant HK. Precise measurement of vertebral mineral content using computed tomography. J Comput Assist Tomogr 1980;4:493-500.
[7] Hangartner TN. The OsteoQuant: An isotope based CT scanner for precise measurement of bone density. J Comput Assist Tomogr 1993;17:798-805.
[8] Davie MWJ, Haddaway MJ. Bone mineral content and density in healthy subjects and in osteogenesis imperfecta. Arch Dis Child 1994;70:331-334.
[9] Zionts LE, Nash JP, Rude R, et al. Bone mineral density in children with mild osteogenesis imperfecta. J Bone Joint Surg 1995;77B:143-147.
[10] Paterson CR, Mole PA. Bone density in osteogenesis imperfecta may well be normal. Postgrad Med J 1994;70:104-107.
[11] Hangartner TN, Gilsanz V. Evaluation of cortical bone by computed tomography. J Bone Miner Res 1996;11:1518-1525.
[12] Miller ME, Hangartner TN. Computed tomography (CT) bone density in children with osteogenesis imperfecta (OI), infants with multiple unexplained fractures (MUF), and controls. Ped Res 1995;37:150A.
[13] Miller ME, Hangartner TN. Increased cortical bone density in adults with osteogenesis imperfecta. Ped Res 1996;39:147A.

Chapter 5

Aggressive (But Gentle) Fracture Management

by Nancy B. White, OT

A person affected with Osteogenesis Imperfecta (OI) spends a considerable amount of time in casts during their lifetime. Therefore, a great deal of time and consideration is spent on the patient with OI. In dealing with a newborn or young child, the family may not be familiar with the fracture treatment process. As the individuals with OI and their families become more knowledgeable, they learn quickly what works well for them. They can become very helpful and it is important to include them in the cast application and removal procedure. Therefore, the more they understand about the importance of aggressive fracture care, hopefully the better the results will be. Over the years of caring for a person with OI, the families can become weary of the repeated trips to the emergency room. They may start treating fractures on their own and not seek out proper medical care. This can lead to more deformities or other complications. It is important the families obtain medical treatment each time a fracture is suspected.

The orthopaedist, orthopaedic technologist, and other health care professionals need to exercise care in the application and removal of a cast. Health care professionals need to become educated about OI and be aware that they can fracture the individual during treatment. Casting and splinting should be administered by an orthopaedic technologist, under the physician's directions, who has been trained in the art and science of cast application and has an understanding of OI.[1]

Temporary Immobilization for Transport

At the initial onset of trauma, it is extremely important to immobilize the injured area for transport to prevent further injury. In an emergency, splints can be made from a number of items from around the house such as newspapers, magazines, cardboard, or a flat piece of wood.[2] These can be secured to the injured area with an ace wrap, towels, or strips of fabric. The splint should not restrict circulation.

Once at the health care facility, a more appropriate temporary splint can be applied for transport to x-ray or surgery. Moving from the emergency room to x-ray or to surgery without adequate immobilization of the fracture can be very traumatic and painful for the patient, and can result in the displacement of previously nondisplaced fractures or further trauma to the extremity.

Nonoperative Methods of Treatment of Fractures

Casts are frequently used for immobilization of a fracture. Correct immobilization is critical in promoting proper healing

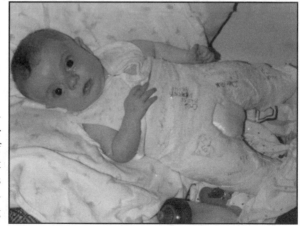

of fractures, preventing displacements, angulation, and rotation, relieving pain, and allowing improved mobility during the healing process. By extending a cast above the proximal joint to below the distal joint of the fracture will ensure adequate immobilization of the site.[3]

The form of treatment required will depend on the particular body part affected and the type of injury. The following is a general look at the different forms of immobilization.

Plaster casts are most commonly used in Primary Casting for the initial treatment of a fracture. Plaster is used because it is pliable and economical.[1]

Secondary casting replaces the primary cast and fiberglass is most often used.[1]

Bracing may be used to maintain a fracture while allowing adjacent joints the freedom for movement. This can reduce rehabilitation time, stimulate bone healing, and prevent disuse atrophy of soft tissues.[1]

Splinting is used to immobilize and maintain a particular position of a bone or joint. Splints are usually constructed of rigid or semirigid strips made of fiberglass, plaster of Paris, or thermoplastic. These are secured to the limb by ace bandages.[1]

Traction is used for the purpose of regaining alignment of a fracture by applying force to the body part. It also can relieve muscle spasms and maintain alignment during bone healing. In skin traction, the pull is applied directly to the skin, not the bones. Skeletal traction is applied directly to the bones by using pins, wires, or screws.[1]

Ideally, after fracture reduction, either a splint or bivalved cast should be applied acutely.[3] If the fracture is stable after reduction, the extremity should be immobilized in the neutral position.[3] Univalving, particularly with a synthetic cast, does not provide adequate flexibility to accommodate swelling of the extremity.[3]

Considerations Unique to Osteogenesis Imperfecta

Immobilization should be kept to a minimum and weight bearing or other functional use of the casted extremity should be encouraged as quickly as possible to prevent further osteopenia. If fractures are allowed to heal without any attempt at alignment or reduction, a progressive deformity or nonunion could result, and the child will lose considerable function.[4]

Children with OI frequently have bowing or other deformities of their extremities which a cast must accommodate. Make note of all bowing in the extremities and curves in the body. An example of this is a child with a femur fracture and an anterior bow of the tibia. A hip spica would be applied after fracture reduction but must be padded well with felt directly over the anterior bow of the tibia. This will cushion the area and reduce the risk of decubitus ulcer.

The patient with OI tends to have contractures develop due to prolonged and frequent casting, so joints should be placed in a neutral position if at all possible. This will help prevent a stiff foot, heel cord contractures, and hip flexion contractures which commonly occur in this patient population. The hips should be positioned at no more than 15-20 degrees of flexion, the knees at 15-20 degrees of flexion, and the ankles at neutral.

With the child with OI, it is important to take extra precautions in the casting of the lower extremities. Since these children break easily, a general rule of thumb is to protect the toes from injury. Numerous families have had their children's toes and/or ankles break while carrying their child immobilized in a lower extremity cast. Use of a full footplate and toe guard during immobilization can help prevent inadvertent fractures.[5] The anterior area of the toes can be left open for checking circulation.

In most patients with OI, you will achieve maximum comfort and minimized muscle spasms with this type of positioning. Positioning of the patient with OI is the most critical aspect of the casting procedure. Also, it is extremely important to follow these patients closely and examine for complications.

Application Techniques

1) Always assemble all of the materials close at hand. Water should be tepid or at the manufacturers specifications.

2) Inspect and cleanse skin surface as needed and apply appropriate dressings.

3) Apply stockinet allowing enough material at each end of the cast to be folded down for finishing the cast. For hip spicas, apply stockinet or Gore-Tex Pantaloon. (See list of cast materials.)

4) Apply cast padding, removing wrinkles. Each turn should overlap the previous one by half the width of the padding.

5) Pad bony prominences adequately with felt. In a hip spica, wrap felt around the entire trunk area, upper medial thighs, anterior iliac crests, and sacrococcygeal region, as well as any bony deformities in the femur, tibia, and foot region. Felt can be applied at the knee and ankle region as you normally would.

6) Recheck positioning.

7) Apply casting tape, overlapping on each turn by half the width of the roll. Incorporate splints in areas requiring additional support.

8) Just prior to setting, gently compress the exterior of the cast with open palms to facilitate molding of the cast to the underlying body contours or as necessary to maintain reduction of the fracture.

9) Turn the ends of the stockinet over the ends of the cast to cushion the margin. Finish out cast with casting tape to secure stockinet in place.

10) Always handle wet cast with the palms of the hands. Handling a wet cast with fingers can put dents in the cast that may cause areas of tissue damage, pressure sores, or nerve palsies.[1]

Hip Spicas

In hip spica, the contour of the chest, back and abdominal area need to be assessed. A towel should be used to allow room for expansion of the abdomen. Allowances must be given for the patient with a barreled chest or short trunk. The patient will become miserable and you could find yourself removing and reapplying a hip spica if it restricts breathing and expansion of the abdomen. At the knee, the supracondyles should be molded well to maintain positioning as swelling subsides.

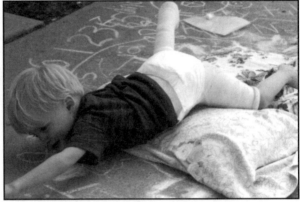

After the pain subsides, children can become surprisingly mobile even in a hip spica.

A well molded hip spica reduces the chances of "settling" in the cast. If settling is suspected it should be addressed immediately. Settling in a hip spica can jeopardize what was accomplished during surgery. Reduction and alignment can be lost and fractures or bowing of the proximal femur can occur. In settling, the child's bottom seems to have changed in the cast and appears to be drooping out of the cast more than previously. A cast which is too loose can lead to settling.

Cast Removal

Once the bone has healed sufficiently, it is time to consider removing the cast. An individual with OI may have delayed healing. Care must be taken when removing the cast not to allow the extremity to dangle. Immediately after cast removal, individuals with OI are very susceptible to refracture. Casts are generally removed with a cast cutter, a cast spreader and bandage scissors.[1] When removing a cast, the patient needs to be told about the equipment and then they need to be reassured that the procedure is safe.

Children are often afraid of being injured by the cast cutter. One way to prepare a child for cast removal is by talking with them about the equipment and letting them touch the equipment. Let them ask any questions they may have and then address these questions on their level. With the cast cutter on, touch it to the palm of your hand to show the child that it is safe. A lot of times the children are afraid of the noise. It would be a good idea to put cotton or ear plugs in the child's ears or have a tape player with headphones to muffle the sound of the cast cutter.

When removing the cast from an individual who has had internal or external fixation, the vibration from the cast cutter can be transmitted to the hardware and the bone. This can be very uncomfortable, even painful in some cases. Keep each stroke of the saw short. When spreading the groove open further use caution not to pull one shell from the other. Alternate spreading the cast from side to side all the way down the extremity. Cut the shell loose from the padding, do not pull apart by hand as it causes jerking of the extremity and can cause a refracture. Remove padding and stockinet gently with bandage scissors.

After the cast is removed, expect to see old, loose, or semi-attached skin. If another cast is not applied before leaving your care, cleanse the skin carefully in order to assess the skin fully for any complications. All findings should be addressed and noted. Cast removal, as application, should be carried out by an orthopaedic technologist that is trained and also knowledgeable of OI. Again, this procedure is under the direction of the attending physician.

Complications and Cast Care Instructions

As health care professionals we must make sure we go over the procedures and the appropriate cast care instructions at the time of each casting. Even the individual with OI and his or her family need to be reminded of the precautions and cast care instructions. There could be a number of factors involved, such as pain, other injuries, or medical problems, etc., that may prohibit them from recalling the proper instructions. Therefore, a written list of precautions and cast care plan is vital in all patients.

With the patient who has OI, it is not uncommon for fractures to not be apparent on the initial x-rays. Some type of immobilization may need to be applied until the injured area can be investigated further. In this case the patient needs to be followed closely and repeat x-rays should be obtained in 3-5 days and again in 7-10 days.

Improper cast application can still be associated with a number of complications.[1] If a cast is too tight, it may result in irritation and pressure that may cause inflammation or ulceration, nerve compression and malfunction, phlebitis, muscle atrophy, fibrous tissue proliferation, and contractures.[1] In severe cases, compartment syndromes can occur, causing progressive vascular compromise and potentially permanent disability.[1]

Fracture angulation, loss of fracture alignment, and loss of apposition may occur as a result of a cast being too loose, either when it is applied or later, after inactivity or reduction of swelling has loosened it.[1] Insufficient padding can cause skin irritation, ulcerations, nerve compression, and phlebitis.[1]

Burns can result from applying cast materials with water temperatures that are too warm and from the crystallization process that produces heat.[1] Burns can also result from excessively high room temperatures and humidity, undersaturated casting tape, applying excessive layers of casting materials, overwrapping the cast with ace bandages, and from using blankets or plastic pillows for support.[1]

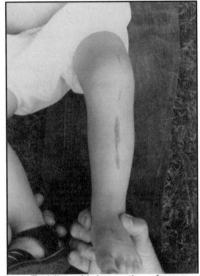

Toddler with lacerations from cast saw.

Even with close attention to treatment the following complications can occur:[2]

Burns	Decubitis Ulcer or Pressure Sores
Cast Syndrome	Dropfoot
Compartment Syndrome	Muscle Atrophy
Constrictive Edema	Pin Tract Infection
Contractures	Thrombophlebitis

It is especially important to investigate complaints thoroughly in the individual affected by OI. Complications that can prolong immobilization can lead to a vicious cycle of fracturing, deformity, osteoporosis, and refracturing.[4] It is critical that we listen carefully to the concerns of the patient and caregiver.

After cast application, precautions and cast care instructions should be explained to the patient and caregiver. This will give the patient and caregiver the opportunity to ask their questions. After going over the instructions, give a copy to the patient and caregiver. Make sure they know how to get in contact with the physician should they encounter any complications. The following has been prepared a guide for your use as is or for you to develop your own set of instructions.

General Precautions for You and Your Cast

Following these precautions will help to assure that you get back to normal as quickly as possible:

1. *Follow your doctor's instructions carefully* regarding physical activity.
2. *Move* fingers or toes frequently to reduce swelling and prevent joint stiffness.
3. *Never Get Cast Wet,* this may cause softening of the cast and irritation to the skin.
4. *Keep dirt, sand, powder, and lotion away* from inside of the cast. Do not pull out the cast padding.
5. *Do not* use oily substances (skin lotion) or powder in or around edges of cast. Oil softens skin and can lead to skin breakdown as well as softening of the cast as it is absorbed. Powder will "cake" under the cast and cause skin breakdown. Rubbing alcohol dries and toughens dry skin, which is the desired effect. It is easier to cure dry skin than pressure areas.
6. Rub the skin under all edges of the cast with rubbing alcohol. Do this four times a day the first week, then as needed to irritated areas.
7. If your doctor fits you with a cast walking shoe, wear it at all times except when sleeping.
8. *Avoid* bumping or knocking the cast against any hard surface.
9. *Do not* use anything to scratch under the cast, since it may break the skin and cause an infection. If itching is a problem, tell your doctor.
10. *Never* stuff cotton, toilet tissue, or Kleenex® under the margin of the cast, since it may fall into the cast, decrease your circulation, and cause serious medical problems. (Watch children that they do not put toys, pencils, crayons, etc. in their cast as this may result in complications.)
11. *Inspect* the cast daily. If it becomes cracked or develops soft spots, contact your doctor.
12. *Elevate* your extremity during the first few days after injury. Elevation helps reduce swelling and discomfort. Also, it may help to apply an ice-pack to the injured area.
13. *Do not* break off rough edges of the cast or trim the cast; contact your doctor.
14. *Never* remove a cast yourself. Your doctor has a special tool to do this.
15. *Contact your doctor* if you have any problems with your cast and especially if you experience any of the following signs or symptoms:
    A. Pain unrelieved by the medication your doctor has prescribed.
    B. Cast feels too snug or tight.
    C. Painful rubbing or pressure develops beneath the cast.
    D. You experience continued coldness or notice whitish or bluish discoloration of your casted limb or unusual odors coming from the cast.

    E. Pain, numbness or a continued tingling of the casted fingers or toes (prolonged irritability of a child).

    F. Cast becomes loose, broken, cracked, or soft.

16. Finally, *use* common sense. Realize you've had a serious injury and protect your cast from damage, so it can protect your injury while it heals.

Doctor's instructions and restrictions regarding physical activities:

_____

_____

_____

_____

Medications: _____

_____

Doctor : _____ Phone Number: _____

Nurse or Orthopaedic Technologist: _____

               Phone Number: _____

Should you have a problem after regular office hours, contact:

_____

               Phone Number: _____

Return appointment date and time: _____

I have received and understand the above information as instructed by

_____ .

             Signature   Date

Summary

A patient affected with OI can be a challenge to any health care professional. Better education will lead to a better level of care for these patients. When referring a patient with OI to another health care professional, it is essential that the proper information be relayed about the patient and OI. It must not be assumed that every health care professional is familiar with OI. With aggressive, but gentle care the results can be successful for the patient and rewarding as well for the health care professional. You may only encounter OI briefly or you may have a patient in your care for years. No matter how often we encounter an individual with OI, we must be knowledgeable of proper cast applications, cast care, cast removal, and OI.

Acknowledgments

I am grateful to my friends and colleagues of the National Association of Orthopaedic Technologists from which I have learned the most about the role that orthopaedic technology plays in patient care for orthopaedic conditions and anomalies.

I am grateful to several health care professionals who encouraged me and offered suggestions to me in writing this manuscript: Drs. J.K. Buck III, L.H. Gerber, D. McKay, W.J. McMahan, and M. Reing. For critical reading of the manuscript, offering valuable comments, guidance and encouragement, the author thanks Dr. Daniel F. Klinar. I am especially grateful to my husband, Anthony L. White, for help in this and all things.

Casting Materials

Cast Cutter (or Saw): electric circular oscillating saw for splitting and/or removing a cast.

Cast Padding: synthetic fiber rolled padding used with fiberglass casts.

Cotton Roll: materials made from cotton that can be rolled as a bandage and acts as a buffer between the skin and plaster material; Webril®.

Felt Padding: thick felt or feltlike material added to the undersurface of a cast on local areas of bony prominences or pressure areas.

Fiberglass Cast: lightweight fiberglass material that is "cured" after being wrapped and exposed to water, which makes the material firm.

Gore-Tex Cast Liner: a unique waterproof, breathable cast padding designed for use with fiberglass casting tape that the patient can get wet.

Gore-Tex Pantaloon: a waterproof, breathable membrane manufactured from polytetraflouroethylene. Pantaloon protects the cast and padding from becoming soiled by urine and excrement when used in body cast or hip spicas.

Moleskin: adhesive, thin, velvetlike material used to smooth edges of casts or to buffer area of excessive skin wear.

Plaster Rolls: gauze roll impregnated with plaster of Paris, which when dipped in warm water (generally 70-75 degrees F) can be applied, rolled smoothly, and molded, becoming hard within ten minutes.

Stockinet: cloth stocking roll used initially in cast applications; comes in many sizes; can be covered by padding followed by firm cast material.

Thermoplastic Casts: heat-sensitive plastics that become soft and malleable when heated and harden again when cooled.

References
[1] Johnson & Johnson Orthopaedics: Cast Applications, 1994, Education Design.
[2] Blauvelt CT, Nelson FRT. A Manual of Orthopaedic Terminology, ed.5, 1994, Mosby -Year Book.
[3] Alpert SW, Yishay AB, Koval KJ, Zuckerman JD. Fractures and Dislocations: A Manual of Orthopaedic Trauma, 1994, Hospital for Joint Diseases Orthopaedic Institute, New York.
[4] Marini JC. Osteogenesis imperfecta: Comprehensive management. Adv Pediatr 1988;35:391-426.
[5] Wu KK. Techniques in Surgical Casting and Splinting, 1987, Lea & Febiger.

6

Spare the Rod, Spoil the Child

by C. Michael Reing, MD

Until a cure is found, the treatment of choice for Osteogenesis Imperfecta (OI) is a carefully orchestrated program of conservative management and timely surgical intervention. For the population with OI, the surgical indications and timing of intercession is far different than for broken bones in the general population. We have progressed from the concept of "don't fix it unless it's broken" to one of timed intervention, individualized to the patient's needs. It is important to understand that the bone involvement varies greatly among patients with OI, even among those afflicted with the same type. For example, the same form of OI can yield bones with large intramedullary canals and cortices "soap-bubbly" in appearance, or it can manifest itself as thin intramedullary canals with more discrete, stronger cortices. Surgical intervention in these cases can be either mandated or contraindicated, depending on several factors which we will discuss. The goal is to determine which patients need surgery, when to perform it, and what type of surgery best suits the individual patient. Equally pressing is making the decision not to intervene surgically.

The mainstay of surgical management in patients with OI is intramedullary rod fixation. The goal of intramedullary (IM) rodding for OI is to correct and prevent the bony deformity that accompanies the disorder. The types of rods available and the techniques for inserting them has expanded significantly. However, the practitioner cannot lose sight of the problems inherent in IM rodding of the long bones of such fragile patients. Despite the improvements in rod technology and surgical techniques, intramedullary rod fixation remains a technically demanding procedure with high complication rates.

Surgical management of Osteogenesis Imperfecta via multiple osteotomies and intramedullary rodding was introduced by Sofield and Millar in 1959. The osteotomies were performed to correct angulation and rotational deformities, after which non-elongating rods were inserted to stabilize the bone. In 1963 Bailey and Dubow introduced an elongating rod now known as the Bailey-Dubow rod (see Figure 1). This rod has retracted ends, much like a curtain rod, with the ends broader than the shaft so that it expands with growth. The concept being that controlled expansion of the rod should eliminate the fractures that occur above and below the ends of non-elongating rods.

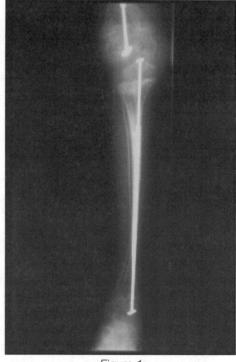

Figure 1.

While widely varying rates of complications have been reported since the 1960's, the most recent studies point to rates in the 70% range for elongating rods and in the upper 50% range for non-elongating rods.[4, 6]

Today, the most commonly chosen non-elongating rods are the Steinmann pin, the Rush rod, and the Enders rod (see Figure 2). Humeral "flex" rods are also used in select circumstances but their acceptance is not as widespread. These non-elongating rods are easier to use than the Bailey-Dubow rod, but have the disadvantage of not expanding to compensate for bone growth, and require reoperation more frequently than the elongating Bailey-Dubow rod.

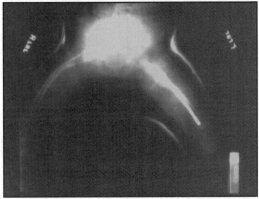

Figure 2.

Other problems inherent in intramedullary rodding systems include: lack of fixation, excessive fixation leading to stress-shielding, difficulty of insertion due to anatomical complications, long bone out-growing non-elongating rods, and failure of elongating rods to extend. If there is a lack of fixation, the rod can migrate through the end of the long bone into the joint or migrate through the soft tissues to the skin. Conversely, the fixation can be rigid; this shields the bone from stress, leads to less bone formation, and, in many cases, bony atrophy, cortical thinning, and resorption of the already weak bone. Rigidly fixed Bailey-Dubow rods are notorious for leaving the patient especially prone to resorption and cortical thinning. If the bone is extremely deformed, multiple osteotomies may be necessary to correct the deformity to a degree that allows insertion of a straight rod. In some cases, the bone is unable to support the insertion of a rod because it is so thin or it possesses almost no intramedullary canal space. When a person with OI reaches the degree of severity such that the bones are so osteoporotic they appear "soap-bubbly" or are barely visible on an x-ray, usually the bone is simply too brittle or too soft to hold a rod of any kind. Non-elongating rods are often outgrown. When this happens, the sections of long bone distal and proximal to the ends of the rod are more susceptible to fracture. Bailey-Dubow and other rods designed to elongate and thereby to correct this problem, do not always do so. Failure to extend may require operative intervention to either repair or replace the rod.

Timing of surgical intervention is extremely important. Luckily it is possible to predict fractures in these patients and to plan preventive surgical intervention. Previous studies have demonstrated that an angulation of forty degrees is the critical point above which fractures will develop (see Figure 3). Thus, it is not a matter of "if" but "when" the fracture will occur. In patients with less than 40 degrees of angulation, a conservative regimen of rehabilitation, muscle strengthening, and bracing as needed, is the best course. In the case of patients with greater than 40 degrees of angulation, there are two choices. The first is to wait until a fracture occurs, then treat both fracture and any deformity with rod fixation. The second is to prophylacticly perform an osteotomy and a rod fixation. It is at this point that the surgeon's judgment and the individual needs of each patient become the primary determining factors.

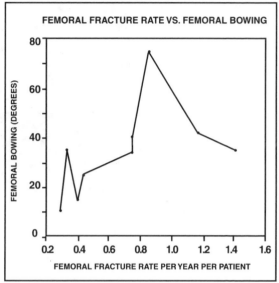

Figure 3.

Once a person has 40 degrees of angulation, it is reasonable to prescribe surgical intervention as the path least likely to obstruct their normal and school schedule.

During the period between electing to perform surgery and the actual surgery, time is "bought" by bracing the patient and enacting protective weight bearing measures via a wheelchair or crutches. If a fracture does occur before the appointed surgery time, the patient should have the full corrective procedure immediately. All too often one sees patients whose fractures were casted and healed before being brought to the operating theatre for definitive treatment. This prolongs the patient's post-operative immobilization and increases the weakening and atrophy of his or her muscles and bones. It is well documented that surgery performed immediately after fracture shortens the rehabilitation period associated with non-operative fracture care and improves the outlook for patient mobility.[2, 3, 6]

In order to best determine which "pre-fracture" patients should have preventive surgery, the treating physician must have knowledge of their family situation and the support they would be receiving pre- and post-operatively. The size and configuration of the bone and intramedullary canal must be scrutinized. Rods have different diameters, and putting a five millimeter rod in a three millimeter intramedullary canal would be an exercise in futility. The physician should also have reasonable expectations of what the operation would accomplish towards improving patient function; it is unfortunate, but some patients with OI will never be functional ambulators. Some fractures and deformities are not amenable to internal fixation in any case. Extreme caution should be exercised in patients with wide intramedullary canals and bones with the "soap-bubble" appearance of thin cortices. While insertion of the rod is not difficult in these patients, it generally will not hold in this type of bone. It has been the experience of this orthopaedic surgeon specializing in OI, and others, that surgical correction of such patients is ill-advised. The majority of this surgeon's attempts with such patients have been singularly unsuccessful.

Once the physician has determined that the patient is a candidate for surgery, he or she needs to be aware of some of the problems unique to this patient population. Anesthesia, nursing, and surgical team members, and recovery room personnel need to be made aware of the fragility of these patients and of the need to take simple measures such as padding their stretchers and the use of appropriate restraints. The small body size of many patients with OI often confuses nursing personnel who tend to treat them as infants rather than young children who are age appropriate in their cognitive development. Anesthesia personnel need to be alerted to the fact that tube size should be gauged by age and head size rather than body size. To be avoided is adherence to the old trick of using an endotracheal tube approximately the size of the patient's pinkie finger. This does not apply to patients with OI and attempts to make it do so will likely necessitate reintubation. Thermal instability is also a problem in patients with OI, and a pseudomalignant hyperthermia with elevated temperature, but without the enzymatic or systemic changes, has been described.

As much as is practical, the patient's surgery should be done with tourniquet hemostasis. When this is not possible, meticulous hemostasis must be maintained. Blood should be available and blood loss carefully monitored; blood volume in patients with OI are body size and weight, rather than age, dependent. A seven year old with OI may only be in the range of 15 to 30 kilograms and therefore would have an intravascular volume of only 1200 to 1600 cubic centimeters. Loss of 120 cubic centimeters of blood in this case would add up to a 10% loss of blood volume. That much blood could be lost in the course of a normal femoral IM rodding, so extreme care must be taken.

During the actual procedure, the surgeon not experienced with patients with OI might be surprised to find a periosteum and soft tissues that yield as much or more resistance than the bone. The surgeon needs to remind him or herself not to squeeze bone clamps tightly and to handle the bone very gingerly so as not to cause unwanted fractures and crush injuries. Unfortunately, flexible reamers with a small diameter are not readily available, but if they can be procured, they make preparation of the intramedullary canal much easier.

Post-operative management of rodded patients is one of the most convincing recommendations for the procedure. Early mobility after fracture fixation is the goal, but one that must be tempered by the surgeon's judgment as to how stable the fixation was at the time of surgery. In general, with intramedullary rods, casts can be removed from patients with OI much more quickly than in patients without OI. This is of critical importance to prevent further degeneration of bone through disuse, joint contracture, and atrophic weakness in the muscles.[1] Intramedullary rods allow speedier rehabilitation of muscles as well, giving the patient as much mobility and self-sufficiency as possible.

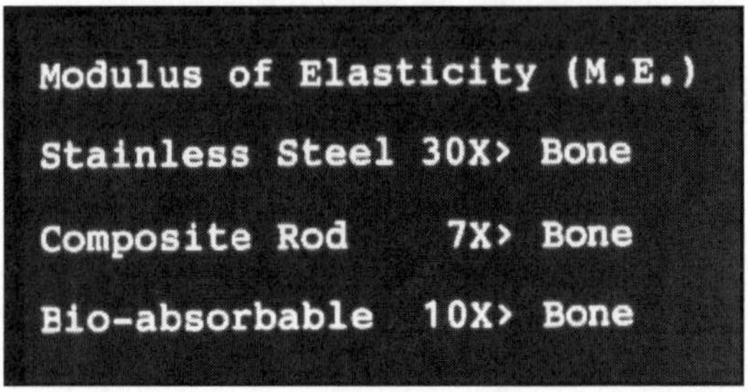

On the horizon of intramedullary rodding in long bones are two developments. In an attempt to address the problem of stress-shielding, testing is underway on composite rods and bio-absorbable rods. The stainless steel

Modulus of Elasticity (M.E.)

Stainless Steel 30X> Bone

Composite Rod   7X> Bone

Bio-absorbable 10X> Bone

Figure 4.

rods currently in use have a modulus of elasticity (ME) 30 times that of bone (ie.: steel is 30 times more rigid than bone; see Figure 4). A rod is expected to be stiff enough to stabilize the fracture and to accept the load across the fracture site. As discussed, this property often leads to cortical resorption and atrophy. Consequently, a search has been ongoing for materials that will stabilize the fracture site and absorb only part of the load – it is essential to proper healing that the bone bear some of the stress across it. Flexible stainless steel plates were examined as a possible solution. The plates eliminated stress-shielding but fractures

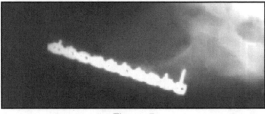

Figure 5.

occurred above, below, and sometimes through them (see Figure 5).[7]

Preliminary animal studies on rods of a composite material with an ME 7 times that of bone have reported only a 4% complication rate.[7] The composite rod is flexible enough to follow the intramedullary canal, thereby easing insertion, and at the same time, it has a permanent memory, allowing it to return to its original shape after stress is applied. All of this not only greatly curtails the incidence of stress-shielding, but it eliminates the need to remove bent or broken rods.

Animal studies on bio-absorbable rods are in early stages. The ME of these rods is 10 times that of bone. While a little of the composite rod's flexibility is lost, the capacity to resorb into the bone after the fracture heals is gained. The process of resorption is a gradual one, allowing the bone to slowly bear more and more of the load across it until it accepts all of it. Problems with the first attempt to study these rods have hopefully been overcome, and trials can progress. Initially, the rods could not be sterilized without structural compromise or upon insertion they absorbed too quickly – before the fracture had fully healed.[7] The clinical trials of the revised bio-absorbable rods are in too early a stage to report on them.

Intramedullary rod fixation and insertion in patients with Osteogenesis Imperfecta can sometimes be a daunting process, and one with a high complication rate. Even in experienced hands, reports are generally of a complication rate around 50% or greater. The bone in patients with OI is easily broken and doesn't hold a rod very well. However, if the physician practices competent patient selection, appropriate timing of surgical intervention, and reasonable surgical technique, the surgery is highly effective. Usually the patient's pain is relieved, his or her deformity is corrected, and he or she is generally able to function at a higher level.[6] Lacking a cure, intramedullary rodding should be regarded as an important tool in the management of patients with Osteogenesis Imperfecta.

Note: The author gratefully acknowledges the assistance of Barbara Keary in the writing of this chapter. Ms. Keary is a pre-medical student at the College of William and Mary who is also a research assistant with Dr. Reing specifically for Osteogenesis Imperfecta.

References
[1]   Binder H, Conway A, Gerber L. Rehabilitation approaches to children with osteogenesis imperfecta: A ten-year experience. Arch Phys Med Rehabil 1993:74:386-90.
[2]   Cole WG. Early surgical management of severe forms of osteogenesis imperfecta. Amer J of Med Gen 1993:45:270-74.
[3]   Engelbert RHH, Helders PJM, Keessen W, Pruij, HEH, Gooskens RHJM. Intramedullary rodding in type III osteogenesis imperfecta. Acta Orthop Scan 1995:66(4):361-364.
[4]   Gamble JG, Strudwich WJ, Rinsk, LA, Bleck EE. Complications of intramedullary rods in osteogenesis imperfecta: Bailey-Dubow rods versus non-elongating rods. J Pediatr Orthop 1988:8:645-49.
[5]   Nicholas RW, James P. Telescoping intramedullary stabilization of the lower extremities for severe osteogenesis imperfecta. J Pediatr Orthop 1990:10:219-23.
[6]   Porat S, Helle, E, Seidman D, Meye, S. Functional results of operation in osteogenesis imperfecta: Elongating and non-elongating rods. J Pediatr Orthop 1991:11:200-203.
[7]   Reing CM. Report on new types of intramedullary rods and treatment effectiveness data for selection of intramedullary rodding in osteogenesis imperfecta. Connective Tissue Research 1995:31(4):S77-S79.

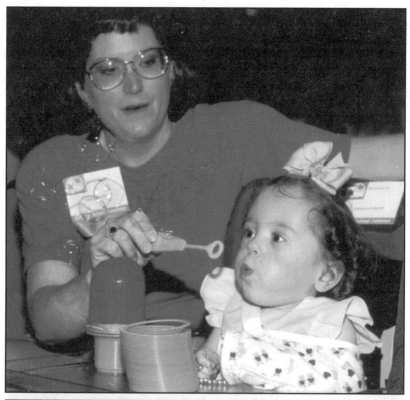

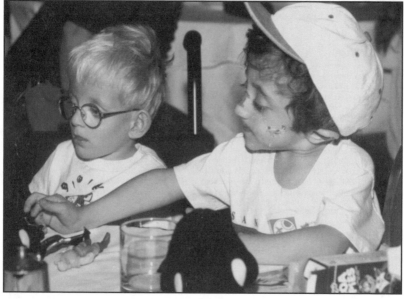

Chapter
Chapter
Chapter
Chapter
Chapter

7

Osteogenesis Imperfecta and Osteoporosis:
Whither the Twain Shall Meet?

By Jay Shapiro, MD

Introduction

One of the common concerns expressed by individuals with Osteogenesis Imperfecta (OI) is whether or not they have developed osteoporosis. Osteoporosis means that bone mass is diminished to the point that fractures may occur with minimal trauma. Confusion arises from the tendency for people to treat these as two independent disorders, rather than from an understanding of the meaning of "osteoporosis" in the context of Osteogenesis Imperfecta. In addition, there is the importance of these two conditions as related to therapy to increase, and thus strengthen, bone mass. From the standpoint of diagnosis, the presence of other osteoporotic individuals without OI in a family expressing mild or Type I Osteogenesis Imperfecta may lead concern for the transmission of a genetic trait where no risk may exist. Finally, the reverse may obtain, that is, the development of age-related bone loss, e.g., postmenopausal osteoporosis, superimposed on a background of Osteogenesis Imperfecta.

Osteoporosis Defined

Osteoporosis most simply defined means less bone.[1] The term is not related to the specific mechanisms by which bone mass is decreased, but

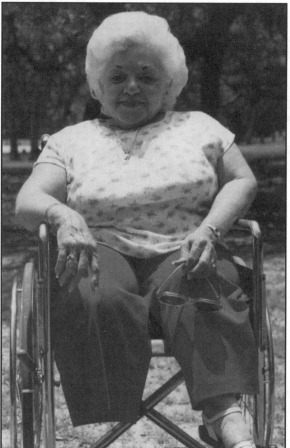

only the magnitude of bone loss as it determines an increased risk of fracture. At any age, fracture risk is best defined relative to the extent of bone loss. Thus, almost all persons with OI are osteoporotic because most persons with OI do not develop normal bone mass at any age. However, it is recognized that occasional individuals with very mild OI have nearly normal bone mass which tends to increase during adulthood.

Advancements in the determination of bone mineral density by dual energy x-ray absorptiometry (DEXA) have made an accurate assessment of fracture risk a readily accessible procedure for women or men of any age.[2] The World Health Organization definition of osteoporosis is a bone mineral density value greater than 2.5 standard deviations below young adult peak bone mass. DEXA measurements are usually reported in terms of bone mineral density (BMD) relative to age-matched controls, a number termed a Z score. In addition, bone mineral density measurements are also calculated relative to young adult peak bone mass which is considered to be age 30 for women and age 20 for men. This number is termed the T score. The risk of fracture is related to a subject's T score, whether determined from the lumbar spine, proximal femur, or forearm. In other words, the risk of fracture is not based on where one stands relative to peers (Z score) but rather on how much bone has been lost from the young adult peak bone mass value (T score). For every standard deviation below the gender matched T score, the risk of fracture increases 2.4 fold. Obviously the same holds for individuals at any age with Osteogenesis Imperfecta. However, the fracture risk may be higher for subjects with OI because not only is mineralization deficient in persons with OI, but the intrinsic organization of bone is defective.

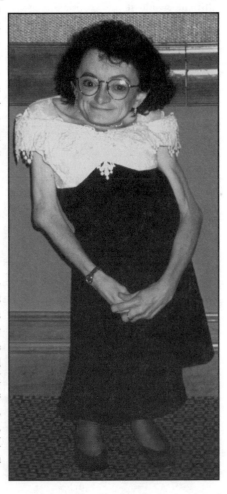

Deficient Bone Formation in Osteogenesis Imperfecta

Research in several laboratories throughout the world has demonstrated that Osteogenesis Imperfecta is the result of many different mutations affecting the synthesis of normal type 1 and type 2 alpha chains of type I collagen. Type I collagen is the major structural protein in bone, tendon, and skin. However, defective synthesis of type I collagen is not the only problem related to the formation of skeletal matrix. Studies in several laboratories have also demonstrated that when isolated bone cells from persons with OI are studied in the laboratory, they demonstrate decreased synthesis of other important components of skeletal matrix; proteoglycans and the matrix proteins osteocalcin and osteonectin are not synthesized in normal quantities by bone cells (osteoblasts) in tissue culture. As a consequence, the normal architecture of bone is disordered in people with OI. Type I collagen fibers are smaller and fewer in number, and the matrix surrounding collagen fibers is also deficient. Normally, calcification occurs at specific sites in the type I collagen molecules. These abnormalities in the formation of normal type I collagen molecules disrupt the process of normal mineralization of these fibers. Thus bone mineral density is also diminished secondary to the synthesis of abnormal type I collagen fibers. Increased fracture risk is the ultimate result of the genetically based metabolic abnormality common to patients with OI.

Osteoporosis in Osteogenesis Imperfecta

Although the primary defect in the formation of skeletal matrix exists in all persons with OI, additional bone loss may occur in patients with OI (as

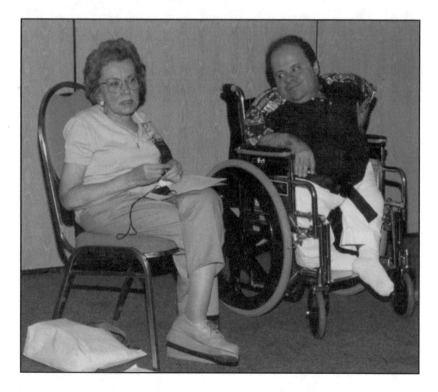

in other individuals) for several different reasons.[3] It is important that these be in mind as patients with OI are evaluated and that diagnostic tests be performed as indicated to be sure that other factors are not contributing to bone loss.[4,5]

Persons with OI may develop any of the more common endocrine disorders that may aggravate bone loss. For example, hyperthyroidism, hyperparathyroidism, and Cushing's disease may develop in patients with OI as in others. In addition, multiple myeloma and various cancers may be the basis for an increase in fracture rate in adults with OI. The development of vitamin D deficiency associated with a fracture in the tibial plateau was observed in a patient with OI who had little sunlight exposure.

Estrogen or estrogen/progesterone replacement is commonly recommended for women following the menopause (see below). Patterson has reported an increase in fracture rate in women with OI following the menopause, assumed to result from the post-menopausal decrease in ovarian hormones.[6] However, an increase in fracture rate probably also occurs in older male patients with OI. The evaluation of an older man with OI should include the determination of testosterone levels, which if low, may be associated with an increase in bone loss.

Prevention and Treatment of Osteoporosis in OI

As presented here, "osteoporosis" is present in almost all persons with OI when defined on the basis of decreased bone mineral density. Prevention strategies, such as weight lifting or walking, may be useful in limiting bone loss in many individuals with OI . Physical therapy is an essential part of the ongoing therapy of a person with OI. At any age, conditioning such as with swimming, walking when possible, and muscle strengthening exercises should be part of every day's routine.

The therapy of osteoporosis in the patient with OI involves two issues: first, therapy to increase the low bone mass that is present at any age as a consequence of the underlying disorder in collagen synthesis, and second, therapy to limit the rate of bone loss that occurs in women and men as a function of increasing age.

The medical literature is replete with a variety of therapies aimed at increasing bone mass in children and adults with OI. There is hardly any agent known to affect bone that has not been tried in patients with OI, including multiple vitamins and hormones. In most reports, only a limited number of patients have been treated, and the results have been inconsistent when tested in larger numbers of individuals. Therapeutic agents currently under investigation include dietary calcium supplements, fluoride, growth hormone, and a second generation bisphosphonate agent, pamidronate. The published data on each of these is limited. As in all older women and men,

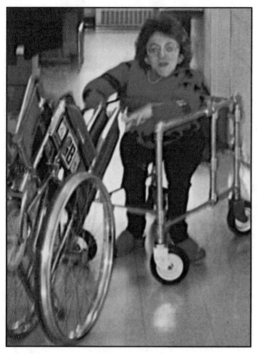

adults with OI should have an adequate calcium intake. The presence of hypercalcuria should be assessed before calcium intake is increased. Bisphosphonate agents are commonly used in the treatment of post-menopausal osteoporosis. Pamidronate administered to children with OI has been reported to produce a significant increase in bone mass. Additional trials with these agents are required to demonstrate their effectiveness for persons with all clinical types of OI and of different ages. Hormone replacement therapy should be considered in all post-menopausal women with OI. In post-menopausal osteoporotic women, hormone replacement therapy is associated with a decrease in fracture rate, both in the lumbar spine and the hip. However, the effectiveness of this has not been critically evaluated in a suitable population of patients with OI. It is not clear whether the osteoblasts in persons with OI are able to respond to the stimulus of estrogen as occurs in the individual without OI, and therefore, a need exists for clinical studies to establish guidelines for hormone replacement in women with OI. Men found to be deficient in male hormones should be treated with testosterone.

Bibliography

[1] Marcus R. The nature of osteoporosis. In: Osteoporosis. Marcus R, Feldman D, Kelsey J, (eds). Academic Press, San Diego, 1996, pp. 647-657.

[2] Johnston CC, Slemenda CW., MeltonLJ, III. Bone density measurement and the management of osteoporosis. In: Primer on the Metabolic Bone Diseases and Disorders of Mineral Metabolism. Favus MJ, (ed). Lippincott-Raven, Philadelphia, 1996, pp. 142-151.

[3] Shapiro JR, Fedarko NS, McBride DJ. Mutations in type I collagen as a cause of a subset of idiopathic osteoporosis. Curr. Opinion Endocrinology and Diabetes. 1994 (1):271-274.

[4] Shapiro, JR. Osteogenesis imperfecta and other defects of bone development as occasional causes of adult osteoporosis. In: Osteoporosis. Marcus R, Feldman D, Kelsey J. (eds). Academic Press, San Diego, 1996, pp. 899-921.

[5] EyreD. Biochemical markers of bone turnover. In: Primer on the Metabolic Bone Diseases and Disorders of Mineral Metabolism. Favus MJ, (ed). Lippincott-Raven, Philadelphia, 1996, pp. 114-118.

[6] Patterson C, McAllison S, Stellman J. Osteogenesis imperfecta after the menopause. New England Journal of Medicine. 1984;(310):1694-1696.

Chapter
Chapter
Chapter
Chapter
Chapter

8

Safe Exercise for Persons With Osteogenesis Imperfecta

By Chester H. Sharps, MD

The benefits of exercise have been well chronicled: better oxygenation, the better sense well-being, increased range of motion, cardiovascular fitness, etc. The ability to achieve the best level of fitness possible, in a safe environment, is the concern of this chapter. Physical fitness will assist persons who have Osteogenesis Imperfecta (OI) with maximizing their overall medical health, mental health, mobility, range of motion, and socialization.

In general, fitness has four specific parts. The first is that of aerobic fitness which is the cardiovascular conditioning of the participant. The second, is the strength for anaerobic conditions. Thirdly, is that of stretching or range of motion considerations which can increase the mobility and quality of movement. The final facet of fitness is the skill for sports specific activity. When developing a safe exercise program that is complete, one needs to consider all of these four aspects.

Osteogenesis Imperfecta is a heterogeneous disorder that at the present time is classified by the Sillence classification. For purposes of this discussion, however, we will use a more functional classification related more to the risk of fractures. Those with severe Osteogenesis Imperfecta are those having a history of multiple fractures with marked deformities of the limbs, short stature, and mobility generally in wheelchairs. Of those with moderate OI, some have had several lower extremity fractures with some experiencing delayed growth. Most are household ambulators, occasionally requiring ambulatory aids. Individuals with mild OI are capable of independent ambulation and only have occasional fractures and normal to near normal height.

Aerobic Fitness

If available, swimming is an ideal aerobic activity for an individual with OI. It not only provides an excellent cardiovascular workout, but also increases flexibility and overall muscular strength and coordination. Gravitational forces are eliminated during this activity, and it is an excellent activity for persons with any severity of OI. If there are no medical contraindications, a swimming program can begin in infancy. Initially, a flotation device to support the neck can be quite helpful. Usually, however, swimming without floatation devices or other physical assistance is an achievable goal.

Difficulty with neck extension is sometimes seen in persons with severe OI and can make the swimming strokes, such as the crawl or breast stroke, impossible. The back stroke is often the only stroke that can be done by persons with severe OI. In contrast, persons with moderate OI can learn the crawl and the breast stroke. Kick boards can be used to assist in the training, as can "noodles" or other types of floatation devices.

Brisk walking for the ambulatory patient or cycling are also excellent activities. Stationary cycling is an activity that can be beneficial to all persons with OI. Tricycling is recommended for most individuals with OI, but bicycling should be individualized for those with moderate or mild impairments. Various recreational mobility aids, such as BIG Wheels® and Safe-T-Trikes® have very wide, low bases of support and are very helpful.

Many persons with mild to moderate OI can participate in "aerobics." There are many commercially available workout videos which can be used. The recommended activities for persons with OI are non-impact to low-impact in nature, such as aerobic walking, step-aerobics, and stairclimbers. For persons who use wheelchairs regularly, aerobic workouts such as Seat-A-Robics® offer cardiovascular fitness and muscle toning. Seat-A-Robics® has videos for children and adults and may be reached at P.O. Box 630064, Little Neck, NY 11363-0064 (Phone number 718-631-4007).

Strengthening

Gaining muscle strength can be very beneficial, not only from the muscle viewpoint, but also from the additional strength that the osseous skeleton obtains from the strengthening of the muscles. The traditional method thought of for building strength would be a weight

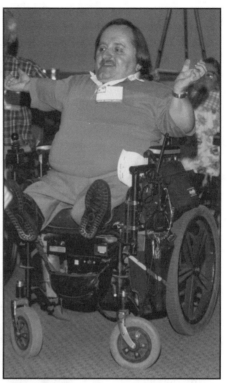

Participant in a Seat-A-Robics® demonstration at the OIF National Conference.

training program with light resistance, which is safe for all persons with OI. Moderate weights can be used by those with moderate and mild OI, and heavier weighted workouts would be reserved for those with mild OI. This can be incorporated in the use of free weights or the use of various weight machines available commercially and also for home use.

Weight training can be done from a sitting or supine position. Programs can be developed to hone in on the areas of specific weaknesses. Workouts should be started with very light weights. The resistance should be very slowly increased with a regular training program. This can be especially useful to strengthen the muscles about the shoulder girdle and also around the pelvis. Stability in these larger areas is very important for continued good mobility. Use of other types of resisted equipment, including exercise equipment or rubber tubing, can be allowed by adherence to the above guidelines. In addition to starting with very light resistance, initial emphasis should be placed on full range of motion of the joints being exercised for sets of ten to twenty repetitions before moving on to higher resistance levels.

Stretching

Stretching is part of any fitness program. Proper length of muscle units around the joints should be obtained with any athlete. Achieving flexibility helps in the fluidity of athletic movement in addition to prevention of injury. Properly warming up prior to beginning a stretching program is an important concept. Slow, gentle, non-ballistic stretching is also recommended.

Sports Specific Activities

In 1983, the American Academy of Orthopaedic Surgeons designed sports participation guidelines for persons with OI. This information serves as a general guideline only as each individual is different.

Table 1 Sports recommended for most persons with OI

Archery
Basketball (wheelchair)
Bowling
Canoeing
Fencing field events
Fishing
Polo (wheelchair)
Rifle shooting
Sailing
Skiing (cross country)
Soccer
Swimming
Table tennis
Tennis
Tennis (wheelchair)
Track
Track (wheelchair)
Tricycling

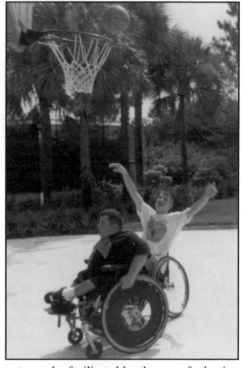

Depending on the special needs of each person, participation in almost all of the sports can be facilitated by the use of adaptive equipment such as using a light weight beach ball or volleyball. Fishing can be facilitated by the use of light weight, but very strong equipment. Electronic reels and rod holders can also be helpful. Wheelchair road racing and wheelchair basketball are also very popular activities which lead to aerobic fitness along with a greater sense of mobility.

Table 2 Sports for persons with mild to moderate OI and should be individualized according to the person with OI

Baseball
Basketball
Bicycling
Diving
Football (touch)
Football (wheelchair)
Golf
Horseback riding
Scuba diving
Skating (roller and ice)
Skiing (downhill)
Softball
Volleyball
Weightlifting

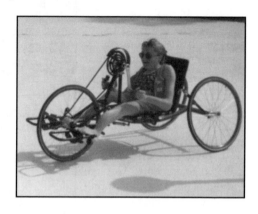

Pre-school and primary grade children with OI usually engage in the motor activities of their peers. The children should be supervised and should be excluded from bodily contact or high impact types of activities.

The lifetime sports listed above, particularly those learned at an early age, can provide an outlet for physical activity and personal satisfaction. Fractures are rarely seen in these sports, particularly archery, bowling, golf, or tennis.

Table 3 Sports in which risks outweigh the benefits

Football (tackle)
Ice hockey
Sledge hockey

One should try to prevent injuries by restricting persons with OI from contact sports, such as wrestling, football, judo, karate, etc. Also, accelerated speed activities, such as skate boarding, wind surfing, etc., should be restricted. Most physicians also caution against tumbling and gymnastics. Long distance running is acceptable, but only for those with mild OI, due to the risk of stress fractures.

Summary

Detailed above are the four aspects of a total fitness program: aerobic conditioning, strengthening, stretching, and skill related activities. Using common sense, combined with certain precautions and adaptive equipment, a program for total fitness can be developed. The physician and/or trainer should be familiar with a number of different sports in order to be sensitive to the likes and dislikes of the participants. After all, if one is engaged in an activity which is tedious and boring, it may not be adhered to for long. Through careful planning and with precautions, the benefits gained through sports and exercise can far outweigh the risks for fractures.

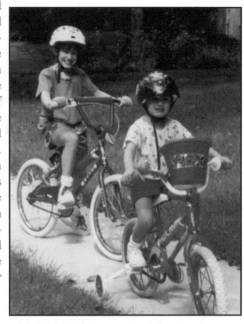

References:

[1] Proceedings of the Winter Park Seminar, "Sports and Recreational Programs for the Child and Young Adult with a Physical Disability," American Academy of Orthopaedic Surgeons, 1983.

[2] Adams R. Physical Activity and Exercise Guidelines for Persons with OI. In: Living With Osteogenesis Imperfecta: A Guidebook for Families. Glauser, HC (ed.) Osteogenesis Imperfecta Foundation, 1994.

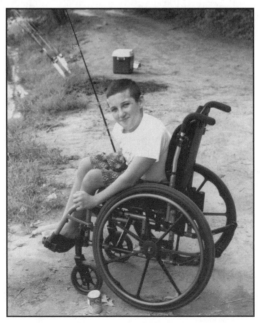

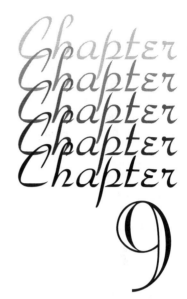

Intrapartum Management

by G.L. Maxwell, MD and J.W. Carlson, DO

Introduction

The intrapartum management of a patient with Osteogenesis Imperfecta (OI) is associated with potential complications which are collectively unique to these individuals. The nonlethal forms of OI (i.e. Types I, III, and IV) vary in severity of illness, making rigid intrapartum recommendations difficult. Intrapartum care must be individualized, taking into consideration the severity of disease known for the mother and anticipated for the fetus. Type II OI often results in delivery of a stillborn or a neonate who subsequently dies soon after birth.[1] Termination of pregnancy should be discussed with the patient having a fetus suspected of inheriting Type II OI. Because of the poor neonatal prognosis associated with Type II OI, the patient may chose to decline cesarean delivery for intrapartum indications during the third trimester. The following discussion pertains to delivery of patients with OI Types I, III, and IV.

Editor's Note: The Osteogenesis Imperfecta Foundation recognizes the sensitive nature of discussions surrounding pregnancies which may result in a baby with Type II OI. Prenatal diagnosis has greatly improved in recent years, but accurately differentiating between OI Types II, III, and IV before birth is often difficult. While the quality of life for children with Type II OI has improved in recent years, there remains a high probability of neonatal or infant death. The decision to continue a pregnancy or not should be made only after the woman has consulted with her family, clergy, and physician.

Discussion

The metabolic abnormalities that occur with OI challenge the obstetrician during labor and delivery. The concern for fractures in the mother and fetus is present throughout labor and delivery. Caution should be utilized in transferring and positioning the mother on an adequately padded bed, to avoid iatrogenic intrapartum injury. In patients with a history of humeral fractures, the procedure of inflating the blood pressure cuff may cause additional fractures or injury.[2] Patients who have OI with a history of pelvic fractures may need to be evaluated for adequate pelvimetry with CT scan, especially in cases involving macrosomic or large for gestational age infants.

Depending on the severity of disease, infants with OI may be at risk for multiple skeletal fractures during labor and delivery. Long bone fractures may require immediate postdelivery stabilization in the otherwise healthy newborn. Skull fractures may be associated with intracranial bleeding that can have adverse neurological sequelae. The risk of fetal skeletal fractures has prompted some investigators to recommend cesarean delivery to all patients with suspected fetal OI.[3] However, several investigators have reported successful vaginal delivery without significant fetal complications in patients with OI Types I, III, and IV.[4-7] Two of these studies advocated cesarean delivery for decreased fetal calvarium mineralization or evidence of fetal fractures and deformations.[5,6] The paucity of published information addressing mode of delivery in patients with OI makes this an unsettled issue. Until further information is available, vaginal delivery is offered to patients without evidence of fetal injury and who have no obstetrical indication for cesarean delivery.

If general anesthesia is utilized in conjunction with cesarean delivery, caution should be implemented by the anesthesia personnel to avoid complications unique to patients with OI. Fasciculations associated with the use of succinylcholine should be minimized, since severe fasciculations may cause fractures in the patient with OI. During intubation, the anesthesiologist should be cautious in extending the neck, manipulating the mandible, and avoiding contact with the dentitia since skeletal fragility makes these structures more prone to fracture.[8] A history

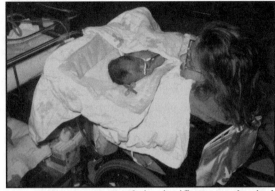

of kyphoscoliosis or pectus excavatum may result in significant mechanical defects of the pulmonary system. Because of the increase in complications associated with general anesthesia in patients with OI, regional anesthesia is advocated.[9]

Patients with OI may have decreased collagen within certain tissues which is usually subclinical, but may be revealed in pregnancy. Young and Gorstein described a case of uterine rupture in a patient with OI who ultimately required cesarean hysterectomy in an effort to control life threatening hemorrhage. The pathological examination of the uterus revealed decreased amounts of collagen within the muscle fibers, indicating that the presence of OI may have increased this patient's chances of uterine rupture.[10] A fetal scalp electrode and intrauterine pressure catheter may allow for the intrapartum diagnosis of uterine rupture and are therefore advocated by some obstetricians.[6] Decreased or abnormal collagen may also lead to weakness of surgical incisions and the risk of postoperative hernia formation.[3,10,11] The use of delayed absorbable or nonabsorbable suture should therefore be considered in closure of uterine and abdominal incisions following cesarean delivery.

Mild hyperthermia and diaphoresis are features which are commonly associated with OI. Increased thyroxine levels may uncouple oxidative phosphorylation causing increased body temperature and oxygen consumption.[12,13] Mild hyperthermia must be distinguished from infection in the intrapartum patient with OI in order to facilitate proper administration of antibiotics. If general anesthesia is contemplated in patients with OI with hyperthermia, agents associated with malignant hyperthermia (i.e. atropine, fluothane, penthane, and succinylcholine) should be avoided in order to prevent exacerbation.[3]

Prolonged bleeding may complicate vaginal or cesarean delivery in patients with OI. The abnormalities in coagulation have been attributed to platelet dysfunction, particularly ADP adhesiveness.[14] A bleeding time is recommended for patients with OI on admission for delivery, and consideration of type and crossmatch of platelets should be performed in patients who experience significant hemorrhage.

Summary

The defect in collagen and the resultant connective tissue abnormalities present the obstetrician with unique problems during delivery of patients with OI. Caution should be utilized in patient transfer and positioning, administration of general anesthesia, closure of surgical incisions, and management of hyperthermia and hemorrhage. Recommendations regarding mode of delivery for patients with OI are currently based on case reports. Until future studies addressing this issue are available, cesarean delivery should be considered for standard obstetrical indications unless sonographic evidence of fetal injury or severe calvarium demineralization exists.

Disclaimer: The opinions contained herein are the views of the authors and are not necessarily the views of the Department of Defense or the United States Army.

References
[1] Bulas DI, Sern HJ, Rossenbaum KN, Fonda JA, Glass RBJ, Tifft C. Variable prenatal appearance of osteogenesis imperfecta. J Ultrasound Med 1994;13:419.
[2] Libman R. Anesthetic considerations for the patient with osteogenesis imperfecta. Clin Ortho Relat Res 1981;159:123.
[3] Roberts JM, Solomons CC. Management of pregnancy in osteogenesis imperfecta: New perspectives. Obstet Gyn 1975;45:168.
[4] Chervenak FA, Romero R, Berkowitz RL, Mahoney MJ, Tortora M, Mayden K, Hobbins JC. Antenatal sonographic findings of osteogenesis imperfecta. Am J Obstet Gyn 1982;143:228.
[5] Kuller J, Bellantoni J, Dorst J, Hamper U, Callan N. Obstetric management of a fetus with nonlethal osteogenesis imperfecta. Obstet Gynecol 1988;72:477.
[6] Carlson JW, Harlass FE. Management of osteogenesis imperfecta in pregnancy: A case report. J Repro Med 1993;36:228.
[7] White CA Osteogenesis imperfecta tarda and pregnancy. Obstet Gyn 1963;22:792.
[8] Cho E, Dayan S, Marx GF. Anaesthesia in a parturient with osteogenesis imperfecta. Br J Anaes 1992;68:422.
[9] Cunningham AJ, Donnelly M, Comerford J. Osteogenesis imperfecta: Anesthetic management of a patient for cesarean section: A case report. Anesth 1984;61:91.
[10] Young BK, Gorstein. Maternal osteogenesis imperfecta. Obstet Gyn 1968;31:461.
[11] Scott D, Stiris G. Osteogenesis imperfecta tarda: A study of three families with special reference to scar formation. Acta Med Scand 1953;145:237.
[12] Solomons CC, Millar EA. Osteogenesis imperfecta: New perspectives. Clin Ortho Rel Res 1973;96:299.
[13] Cropp GJA, Myers DN. Physiological evidence of hypermetabolism in osteogenesis imperfecta. Pediatrics 1972;49:375.
[14] Hathaway WE, Solomons CC, Ott JE. Platelet function and pyrophosphates in osteogenesis imperfecta. Blood 1972;39:500.

Case Study: Pregnancy in Woman With OI Type III/IV

by Garrett H. C. Colmorgen, MD

SMS is an 18 year old, Gravida 2 Para 0010, with known Osteogenesis Imperfecta Type III/IV who presented for her first prenatal visit at approximately eight weeks gestation. The patient's past history is positive for multiple fractures and surgery including fusion of the cervical, thoracic, and lumbar vertebrae. She also had undergone placement of femoral and tibial intramedullary rods. She has had approximately four transfusions. Her past obstetrical history is positive for a first trimester spontaneous abortion prior to this pregnancy.

On physical examination, the patient was found to be of short stature with a height of four feet, one-half inch, and a pre-gravid weight of 35 kilograms. Significant findings included evidence of multiple fractures of the extremities. Her back appeared to be "rigid." Scars from multiple surgical procedures were evident. As a result of femoral and tibial surgery, the patient was felt to have normal strength and essentially normal range of motion. The patient was unable to tolerate a vaginal speculum examination due to the deformities of her pelvis. Bimanual examination revealed evidence of a contracted pelvis: the diagonal conjugate was eight centimeters, spines were prominent, the sacrum was anterior, and the pelvic arch was narrow.

Prenatal Course:

Early in her pregnancy, the patient had molecular studies performed. She was informed that prenatal diagnosis was available via chorionic villus sampling, but not by amniocyte analysis. At her first prenatal visit, the patient expressed an interest in prenatal diagnosis, but she ultimately decided against it. At fifteen weeks gestation, the patient underwent a targeted ultrasound examination that was normal except for a placenta previa. The patient then transferred care to a midwifery clinic. She returned to the major medical center at approximately 28 weeks gestation due to the findings at the time of a targeted ultrasound examination. The fetus was found to have shortening of all of the

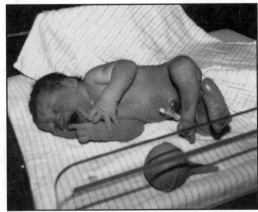

limbs and evidence of fractures. The fetal femurs were bowed bilaterally. Hydramnios was noted. The patient was found to have gestational diabetes (Class A1). At 32 weeks gestation, the fetus was again found to have evidence of bowing and healed fractures. At 35 weeks gestation, the patient was admitted due to preterm labor. The patient underwent amniocentesis to evaluate the fetus for evidence of pulmonary maturity. The L/S ratio was 1.3/1. The patient agreed to undergo a therapeutic amniocentesis due to the hydramnios. Unfortunately, the procedure was terminated after only 300 milliliters of amnionic fluid was removed due to the pain experienced by the patient. Nonetheless, the patient's contractions resolved, and she was discharged to home at bed rest.

Labor and Delivery:

At 38 weeks gestation, the patient presented in active labor. Because of the contracted pelvis, the patient was delivered by cesarean section of a 3050 gram female with Apgar scores of seven at one minute and eight at five minutes. Because of the strong suspicion that the baby was also affected with OI, she was transferred to the Neonatal Intensive Care Unit for further evaluation.

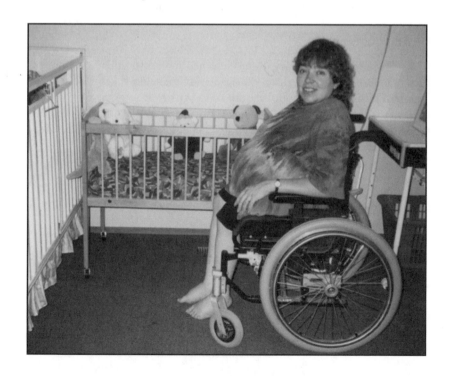

Chapter 10

Making the Diagnosis

by Peter H. Byers, MD

Osteogenesis Imperfecta (OI) is a clinical continuum in which severity ranges from lethal in the perinatal period to such a mild presentation with occasional fracture that the diagnosis often is not suspected. Given this spectrum, what clinical, biochemical, and molecular genetic tools are available to help the clinician make the diagnosis and then to provide appropriate information for the affected individuals and their family members? It should be remembered that the comprehensive care for children and adults with OI involves many specialties: the primary care practitioner, the geneticist, the orthopaedist, and the rehabilitation specialist. Diagnosis and care are not complete until the family has seen each of these people and arrangements have been made for ongoing care.

The Clinical Diagnosis of OI

Despite major advances during the last several years in the understanding of the molecular basis of OI, the diagnosis is almost always considered first on clinical grounds. The principal guiding features used to make the diagnosis of OI, and then to determine the type of OI, are fractures out of proportion to the injury, the presence of blue sclerae and/or dentinogenesis imperfecta (DI), and additional features of connective tissue disorders that include increased joint laxity, some increase in bruising, and short stature. On clinical grounds, the question of OI in a patient arises in several circumstances: the presentation of a child with fractures, the recognition of blue sclerae in the child, and the recognition of bony abnormalities during routine ultrasound surveillance of pregnancies. Each of these needs to be considered separately.

OI Type II. The diagnosis of OI Type II (the perinatal lethal form) generally occurs at one of two points: during routine obstetrical ultrasound studies early in the second trimester (usually around 16 weeks of gestation)

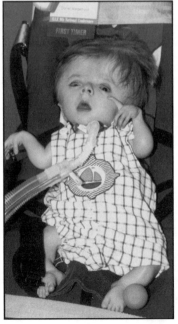

or at birth. Skeletal abnormalities on the ultrasound studies generally raise the issue of OI as a diagnosis. Although most often completed around 16 weeks gestation, the studies can be done as early as 14 to 15 weeks if there is increased risk for a pregnancy with OI Type II. In the absence of sonographic surveillance, the birth of a child with femoral bowing and compression, bowing of the tibias, or soft calvaria is the usual impetus to consider the diagnosis of OI. Most of the children recognized at birth are likely to have either the most severe form of OI (Type II, or the perinatal lethal form) or Type III OI (also known as the progressive deforming variety). Because both usually result from new dominant mutations in one of the genes of type I collagen, a family history is generally "unremarkable" although parental mosaicism (that is, a small number of cells that carry the altered allele on the background of most cells that carry the normal allele) can presage recurrence in the family. It is the physical examination and the radiologic picture that confirm the diagnosis of Type II OI. These infants have soft skulls, the nose is often beaked, the sclerae are often dark blue or grey, the upper and lower arms are generally short, the thighs are generally very short, and the lower legs are bowed in an anterior posterior direction. The lower limbs are carried in a "frog-leg" position (external rotation at the hips and flexion at the knees), and the chest is generally very small. When x-rays are examined, the skull is markedly deficient of mineralization, and the ribs are generally broad with a "ribbon-like" appearance or may be thin with multiple "beads." The long bones are short and deficient in mineralization. The femurs are short and appear compressed ("like an accordion"), and there is bowing of the bones of the lower limbs. Because of the small chest size, the respiratory rate of the baby is generally elevated. The infants are often cyanotic, and demise within a few hours is the general rule, though some have lived for several years.

The diagnosis is generally suspected on clinical grounds with corroboration coming from the radiological picture. The diagnosis can be confirmed on biochemical grounds by analysis of the collagens synthesized by cultured dermal fibroblasts (or from most other tissues taken at autopsy), and the molecular defect can be identified by analysis of the type I collagen genes from those cells. At present, the last step does not add to the diagnosis, but does permit evaluation of the parents for mosaicism, which is valuable for future prenatal diagnostic studies (see below). On clinical grounds, the usual differential diagnosis is limited to other lethal dwarfing conditions that include thanatophoric dysplasis (due to new dominant mutations), hypophosphatasia (a recessively inherited disorder), and achondrogensis (either a new dominant disorder or a recessively inherited disorder, depending on the type). These can be differentiated by the experienced pediatric radiologist and by biochemical or molecular genetic studies.

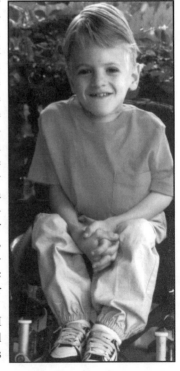

OI Type III. Infants with OI Type III are usually recognized in the perinatal period because of fractures and deformities noted at birth. Clinically, these infants generally have a normal feel to the skull, the sclerae are often grey or blue but not generally dark, the chest may be slightly small, and the upper legs are slightly short while the lower legs are generally bowed. Upon radiological examination, the skull may appear slightly thinned. The ribs are generally thin, and there may be frank new fractures or evidence of healing fractures. The tibias are generally bowed while the fibulas may be very thin. Again, biochemical studies of the collagens synthesized by cultured fibroblasts can confirm a diagnosis of OI, but currently, the type of OI depends on clinical and radiographic criteria. The differential diagnosis is limited with uppermost considerations given to hypophosphatasia and campomelic dysplasia (characterized by bowing and, in some, reversal of the phenotypic from the genotypic sex). OI Types II and III may be referred to as the congenita forms of OI in the older literature and in the current orthopaedic writings.

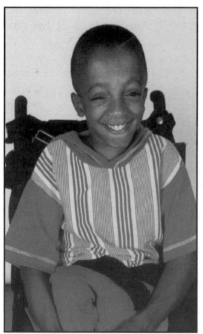

OI Type IV. The diagnosis of OI Type IV often is not considered in the newborn period unless in utero fractures have been noted relatively late in gestation (at more than 24 weeks) or unless fractures occur in the perinatal period. At birth, these infants are generally of average length, usually do not have fractures, and their sclerae are often of near normal hue or compare with the typical bluish color of a newborn's sclerae. The diagnosis is often delayed until a fracture which may occur as the child begins to stand, walk, and fall or until the teeth erupt and opalescence of the dentin can be recognized. Once suspected, the diagnosis of OI can be confirmed by analysis of the collagens synthesized by cultured dermal fibroblasts. In children or adults with mild forms of OI Type IV, the diagnosis may not be suspected until after several fractures have occurred, especially if stature is near average (as it can be) and if the dentinogenesis imperfecta is not present.

OI Type I. The diagnosis of OI Type I typically occurs about the time children start to walk (and fall), in the absence of a prior family history, or in the newborn period if the family history is known and the frankly blue sclerae are recognized. These children are generally of average stature and infrequently have dentinogenesis imperfecta. Again, the diagnosis can be confirmed by the study of cultured fibroblasts. In this instance, OI Type I can be distinguished from the other forms of OI because the cells make about half the normal amount of structurally normal type I collagen. In all the other forms of OI, the cells make some normal and some abnormal collagen molecules.

Prenatal Diagnosis of OI

Prenatal diagnosis of OI usually becomes an issue in two situations: a pregnancy following the birth of an infant with OI to unaffected parents and a pregnancy where one of the parents has OI. Prenatal diagnosis is generally done with one of several questions in mind:

1.) Is the fetus affected?

2.) Should decisions be made about continuation versus termination of pregnancy?

3.) Will the knowledge that the fetus is affected alter the perinatal decisions concerning the mode of delivery?

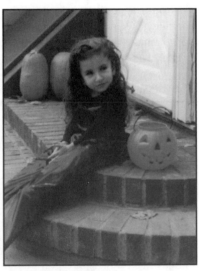

Some considerations are appropriate when pondering each of these issues. First, the recurrence risk following the birth of a first child with a dominantly inherited form of OI to parents who are not themselves affected is generally small – on average three to four percent (3-4%). Usually, the affected child born to unaffected parents has a new mutation, but the recurrence in multiple children of a family reflects parental mosaicism for the mutation. Mosaicism occurs when the mutation took place in a parent during his or her embryonic life, but only some cells, including the germ cells, carry the mutation. If one parent is determined to be mosaic, then the risk of recurrence is generally higher than the background risk, but would not exceed 50% (50% recurrence risk occurs when all germ cell progenitors carry one copy of the mutation bearing chromosome). The prenatal diagnostic strategy needs to be targeted to the specific form of OI (see below).

Second, decisions about pregnancy termination are obviously not easy and are subject to a variety of pressures and considerations. Although both the physician and family members may be comfortable ahead of time with their perceptions of what will be done in the event that OI is present in the fetus, these decisions may change with time and all should be aware that prenatal diagnostic studies do not commit the family to any specific course of action.

Finally, it is not clear that one mode of delivery makes a difference for the fracture rate in children with milder forms of OI, or in the survival for children with Type II OI. Indeed, decisions concerning the mode of delivery generally reflect the presence of the more common obstetric problems (breech lie, fetal distress, etc.) rather than the concern for OI.

There are four approaches to the prenatal diagnosis of OI: ultrasonography, protein based studies of cultured chorionic villus cells, analysis for the specific mutation in the family, and linkage studies. Each of these depends on the status of knowledge about the cause of OI in the family. The risk for pregnancy loss is quite different with each of these procedures.

Ultrasonography. Increasingly common with the use of routine obstetrical studies is the identification of a fetus with bony abnormalities, particularly short bones and the suggestion of fracture. In most instances, such a diagnosis occurs in the absence of a family history of fetal wastage or abnormality, and the issue is the nature of the skeletal abnormality. Amniocytes cannot be used to study the collagens synthesized because they do not make the appropriate molecules. Biopsy of the placenta may be helpful, but the growth of cells and the diagnostic studies take about three to four weeks. Thus, if the sonographer is uncertain of the diagnosis, referral to a tertiary care center (often a university medical center with experienced sonographers) is the single most useful approach to clarification of the differential diagnosis. The fetal skeleton is abnormal by 16 weeks in OI Type

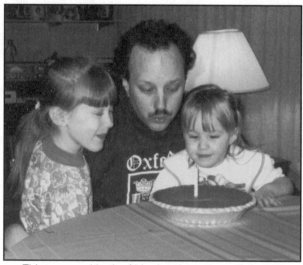

This man and both of his daughters have Type I OI.

II, but may not be abnormal until 18 weeks in OI Type III, and is often not abnormal in OI Types I and IV. There is little, if any, increased risk for pregnancy loss associated with the procedure.

Biochemical Studies of Cultured Chorionic Villus (CVS) Cells. In contrast to amniocytes, chorionic villus cells synthesize the same collagen molecules as skin and bone cells. Type I collagen is the major structural protein of bone and the protein in which the vast majority of abnormalities detected in persons with OI are found. Thus, if abnormal collagens are synthesized by fibroblasts from a family member with OI, then CVS cells can usually be used to determine if a fetus at risk is affected. The biopsy is generally done at about 10 weeks gestation. The cells take about 10 days to grow, and the diagnostic studies are generally completed in an additional 10 days. Thus, diagnostic information can be available by 13 to 14 weeks gestation, commensurate with the timing of sonographic diagnosis of OI Type II, but far sooner than the diagnosis of OI Types III or IV could be made by ultrasound. Such studies are only effective for the types 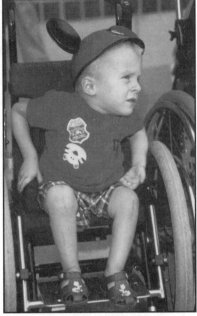 of OI in which abnormal molecules are made (OI Types II, III, and IV), but not OI Type I because of the difficulty with quantitation of the amount of type I collagen synthesized by cultured cells. Chorionic villus biopsy generally presents a risk of one to two percent (1-2%) pregnancy loss for the procedure itself when done by experienced centers.

Specific Molecular Diagnosis. During the last decade, the specific mutations in more than 200 individuals/families with OI have been identified. There are some mutations that have been recognized in more than one family, but the majority of those identified so far are unique to the family in which they were discovered. Although this reflects the difficulty in molecular diagnosis, the other side of the coin is that when the information is available, it can be used both for prenatal diagnosis and for the identification of other people in the specific family who are also affected. These studies require a small amount of DNA from the target individual and can include any cell in the body. If the mutation is known, it takes only a few days to isolate the DNA from the fetus in question, or a fmily member at risk, and to do the testing. The risk for pregnancy loss as a consequence of amniocentesis done at 16 weeks gestation may be as little as 0.5% above the usual rate of loss for that specific period. The more timely CVS sampling is usually done at 10 weeks gestation.

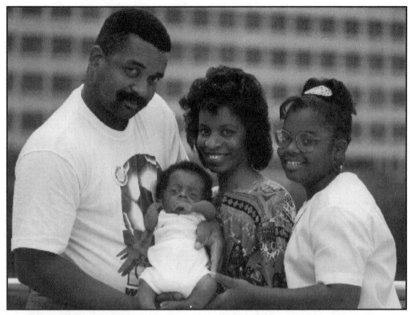

Linkage Studies. In a family, the diagnosis of OI can often be confirmed by tracing the altered copy of the gene through the family. When the mutation is known, this is straightforward and readily understood. It is possible, however, even in the absence of the specific mutation, to track the chromosome that bears the mutation through the family using common variations in the two causative genes to trace the copies through the family. This procedure, known as doing linkage or segregation studies in the family, requires that blood be drawn from all affected and unaffected members of the family. DNA is extracted from the blood, these variations are analyzed, and their transmission through the family determined. While often feasible, the family size may not be sufficient to come to the diagnosis. The laboratory in which the studies are to be done should be consulted before blood is drawn.

Child Abuse and OI

It has been proposed that almost half a million children are physically abused each year, and more than a third of those suffer fractures. Because abusing parents may themselves have been abused as children, a "family history of fractures" is often obtained. The diagnosis of non-accidental trauma relies on several aspects of the presentation – a typical pattern of fractures, inconsistency of the described events with the extent of injury, and the absence of clinical features that suggest an alternative diagnosis. The question of OI is often raised in these circumstances. The search for a good diagnostic discriminatory test has often led parents, physicians, social workers, and officers of the court to ask for diagnostic skin biopsies to be performed. The expected outcome in these situations is that the studies of a child who has been abused will always be within normal limits and those of a child with OI will always be abnormal. Two issues cloud this outcome. First, biochemical studies of collagen biosynthesis and structure identify about 90% of children known to be affected with OI on clinical grounds. Second, children with OI can be abused so that the finding of biochemical abnormalities does not exclude the possibility of abuse.

Currently, the cost of direct molecular testing (estimated at about $2000 per study) is too high to be used realistically in this setting. The cost of biochemical studies is about $750 per study. It remains clear that careful and conscientious clinical evaluation is probably the most efficient means for management in this setting.

Issues in the Biochemical and Molecular Diagnosis of OI

It is important to remember that the biochemical and molecular genetic studies provide confirmation of the clinical diagnosis of OI, and can distinguish the mild Type I OI from the more severe deforming varieties. The biochemical studies confirm the diagnosis of the more severe forms, but often do not distinguish between the milder forms of OI Type IV and the more severe progressive deforming varieties of OI Type III. Even the molecular genetic studies do not yet clearly distinguish between the types unless precisely the same mutation has been identified in another individual. Even

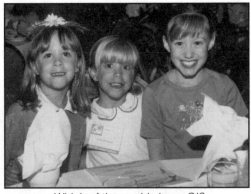

Which of these girls have OI?
(see answer below.)

then, intrafamilial variability can be marked, and interfamilial variation can be considerable. Both biochemical and molecular diagnostic studies are very important in the context of prenatal diagnosis because these studies are difficult to complete unless the abnormalities are known.

ANSWER: The girl in the middle does not have OI. Her sister (left) and her cousin (right) both have Type I OI.

Biochemical studies of collagens synthesized can be performed on cultured skin fibroblasts as well as a number of other tissues, including foreskin taken during circumcision. Most molecular diagnostic procedures currently start with cultured cells and use the mRNA for the collagen genes to construct DNA copies which are then analyzed for mutations. Direct analysis of genomic DNA (taken, for example, from white blood cells) is feasible and such diagnostic strategies are now being utilized.

Additional Reading

Wenstrup RJ, Willing MC, Starman BJ, and Byers PH. Distinct biochemical phenotypes predict clinical severity in nonlethal variants of osteogenesis imperfecta. Am J Hum Genet 1990;46:975-982.

Byers PH. Osteogenesis Imperfecta. In: <u>Connective Tissues and its Heritable Disorders</u>. Royce PM, Steinmann B. (Eds). Wiley-Liss, New York, 1992, pp. 317-350.

Byers PH. Disorders of collagen structure and synthesis. In: <u>The Metabolic and Molecular Bases of Inherited Disease</u>. Scriver CR, Beaudet A, Sly W, Valle D. (Eds). McGraw-Hill, New York, 1995, pp. 4029-4078.

Steiner RD, Pepin MG, Byers PH. Studies of collagen synthesis and structure in the differentiation of child abuse from osteogenesis imperfecta. J Pediatr 1996;128:542-547.

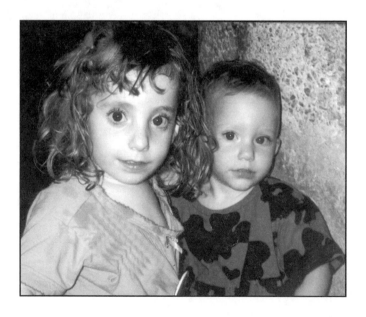

Chapter
Chapter
Chapter
Chapter
Chapter

11

Care of the Newborn With Severe Osteogenesis Imperfecta

by Robert D. Steiner, MD and Anna August, MD

The newborn period for the parents of a child with Osteogenesis Imperfecta (OI) is a critical time. It is during this period that the family often learns of the diagnosis and goes through the initial process of grieving for the loss of the "normal child" they expected. In addition, many of these children are sick and parents must face the additional stresses that accompany having an acutely ill child. They are forced to accept the diagnosis of an often debilitating and sometimes fatal condition, and remain coherent enough to be involved in decisions about the care of their child. Not uncommonly, decisions about continuing life support measures need to be made early, before the family has had time to comprehend what the disease involves and the longer term implications of continuing supportive measures. Guilt, sadness, depression, and anger are common emotions experienced by these parents, although not always outwardly apparent. Attempts should be made to minimize the emotional trauma to the family by involving caretakers with experience with this condition, while providing the appropriate care to the baby. This would typically include a medical geneticist, neonatologists experienced in the care of sick newborns, and nurses and social workers who can address the needs of the family.

Prenatal Decision Making

With recent advances in prenatal diagnostic techniques, an increasing number of parents may learn that their child has OI prior to birth. A screening ultrasound, which may or may not detect OI depending on timing and level of detail, is performed routinely during most pregnancies. For parents who have had a previous child with OI, detailed ultrasound examination looking specifically for OI is offered. Chorionic villous sampling done at 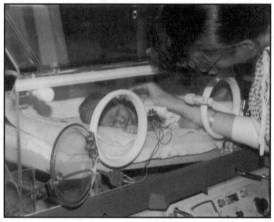 9-12 weeks gestation may allow early diagnosis by genetic or biochemical techniques if the affected child was found to have a biochemical or genetic defect of collagen or collagen genes. (See chapter 10 for further discussion of diagnosing.) With early diagnosis, the family can then proceed down the path that they choose. This may include delivering the infant at a center that has a Newborn Intensive Care Unit (NICU) on site, where experts in both medical genetics and newborn care are readily available to attend to the infant, confirm the diagnosis, and help the family make appropriate decisions for the child. Other families may choose to carry the child to term but prefer no aggressive measures to keep the baby alive, while others will choose to terminate the pregnancy. There is no "correct" approach to this situation, and the family should be supported in whatever decision they make. Despite a family history of OI, many families will make an informed decision not to have prenatal testing, and that should also be supported.

Editor's Note: The Osteogenesis Imperfecta Foundation recognizes the sensitive nature of discussions surrounding pregnancies which may result in a baby with Type II OI. Prenatal diagnosis has greatly improved in recent years, but accurately differentiating between OI Types II, III, and IV before birth is often difficult. While the quality of life for children with Type II OI has improved in recent years, there remains a high probability of neonatal or infant death. The decision to continue a pregnancy or not should be made only after the woman has consulted with her family, clergy, and physician.

Prenatal testing also allows for the learning process and in some cases the grieving process to begin before birth. The family can avoid the difficult task of explaining to family and friends after birth that the child has a condition which is often disfiguring or fatal. Some parents feel it is easier to explore these issues prior to birth when there are not all the expectations and commotion commensurate with a new birth. If the diagnosis is not known prenatally, health care workers at the delivery may not recognize the diagnosis immediately or the dismal prognosis which OI Type II portends and therefore may feel obligated to do everything they can to keep the baby alive. This often involves separating the baby from the parents at a critical time when the optimal course may be to let the baby stay with the family and die peacefully in their arms. In addition, in the case of mild OI, health care providers at the delivery of a baby diagnosed prenatally will be cognizant of the need to use care in handling the infant to prevent fractures.

Resuscitation

Once the child with OI is born, the course followed next depends on the severity of the condition, which can vary tremendously. In persons with Type II and severe Type III OI, difficulty breathing is often present immediately after birth and often the infants will die rather quickly without aggressive resuscitation. Intubation (placement of a plastic tube in the trachea) and mechanical ventilation by a respirator are often required to maintain the child, and frequently the decision of whether or not to proceed with these heroic measures must be made within minutes of birth. If these decisions can be discussed beforehand and appropriate plans made, the delivery room becomes a much more peaceful environment. Asking the family to make decisions about resuscitation of an infant in the delivery room with no previous discussion of the condition is not tenable. Decisions about resuscitation are made by the care team in conjunction with the family. It is important not to put the tremendous burden of determining course of action on the family, but rather to help them understand the issues so that their feelings can enter into the decision making process. These decisions must be individualized based on each family's beliefs and desires, as well as the prognosis for the baby. We must keep in mind that the developmental and intellectual prognosis in OI is good, and most often it is the skeletal abnormalities of the chest that create a life threatening situation and are often impossible to overcome.

When families have decided against resuscitation, emphasis should be placed on letting the family hold the infant and keeping the baby comfortable. Should the decision to aggressively resuscitate a child with OI be made, it is very important to be extremely gentle with each procedure. Intubation should be performed by the most experienced person. The head should not be hyperextended but kept in a neutral position, the mouth should be gently opened with a finger, the laryngoscope inserted carefully, and the trachea intubated. Intravascular access (placement of an IV) can be obtained most gently through an umbilical vessel rather than attempting peripheral intravenous catheter placement. When placing monitor leads and moving the infant between beds, slow, deliberate movements will cause the least trauma. Everything should be prepared for the move ahead of time, so that it can be accomplished smoothly. Care should also be used when obtaining x-rays, and any blood work should be obtained, if possible, from an umbilical catheter and not by heelsticks or venipuncture.

Parent/Child Bonding

The Newborn ICU can be an intimidating and frightening place and support should be given to the families, as well as privacy for them and the baby if possible. For infants that must be transferred away from the parents for care, time must be taken to let the parents see and touch the baby, and even hold the infant if possible before transfer. Comprehensive care in the NICU is best delivered with a team approach including individuals from pediatrics, medical genetics, orthopaedics, nursing, physical therapy, occupational therapy, and social work. The neonatologist, a newborn specialist, is the leader of the team. Parents expecting a child likely to spend time in the NICU are encouraged to take a tour of the unit before the child is born to become familiar with the surroundings and the staff.

Parent/child interactions should be interrupted as little as possible with any sick child and should be encouraged even if the child is in the NICU or dying. Infants with OI who are dying should be allowed to spend as much time with the parents as possible, with as much privacy as possible. When the prognosis is poor, there is no need to keep the parents from holding the infant for fear of bone injury. The benefit to parents from holding the baby far outweighs the risk of any further bony damage. If the issue of comfort is raised, then narcotics can be administered to the infant. Once the decision to withdraw heroic support is made, the wires, tubes, and lines that connect the infant to monitoring devices, ventilators, and intravenous fluids, should be removed so the child can be held and comforted.

Some parents find it helpful for other family members or close friends to be present or available for much-needed support during this time. This period of bonding is invaluable; nothing can replace the bonding that takes place when a parent holds his/her child for the first time. The time spent with the baby will be remembered and cherished. As with any situation where we cannot improve the outcome for the baby, we can make the situation less traumatic for the family, and try to ensure some pleasant memories with their child. With time, it is the special moments holding their baby, or having family see the child, that are remembered most. For parents that have lost a child with OI or have a child with OI, it is important to offer them the opportunity to speak with other parents who have had similar experiences. The OI Foundation is an extremely valuable resource especially in that regard.

Often babies with severe OI may not look normal, and not infrequently the family has difficulty looking at a baby who appears "different". Most parents look past these problems and are able to bond immediately to their child. For those parents that appear to be having difficulty, it is important to encourage them to see and hold the baby, and explain why the abnormal features are present. Families with children with less severe OI are not faced with the same issues as those with severe OI. Still, they have a child with a chronic disease which will require adjustment and they need as much support as the other parents. Those with relatives with OI, may have had enough exposure to affected individuals that having a child with OI takes less education and adjustment. Other families may seem devastated when informed of the diagnosis, and health care providers should respond to a family's needs and the messages they are giving. Most families will benefit from learning as much as they can about OI. In many cases it is fear of the unknown and a feeling of helplessness that creates much of their stress. Through education, we may be able to allay many of their concerns and fears.

Practical Handling Tips

There is surprisingly little information available in the form of books, pamphlets, or journals to parents and health care providers on the practical aspects of caring for a newborn and young infant with OI. Parents should not assume that health care providers are knowledgeable about OI since most pediatricians will never care for an infant with OI during an entire career. Common sense is the guiding principle in caring for children with OI. A good rule of thumb for health care providers is that management of OI patients during the neonatal period does not differ significantly from that of infants of similar birth weight with the exception of the special handling necessary to avoid fractures. Also, special attention should be paid to fluid status in the very small infant with OI since fluid loss through the skin can be excessive. Parents with children who have OI learn quickly how to best care for these infants. For this reason, health care providers should be open to parents' suggestions and respect the knowledge they have acquired by caring for their children.

We have outlined below a series of specific recommendations for care of the infant with OI. Most of these recommendations are made with the caveat that few of these procedures have been studied to prove efficacy. Many come from parents of children with OI based on anecdotal experiences. Others represent the authors' suggestions based on their experiences and hopefully adhering to the common sense principle. OI is an extremely variable condition and some infants are much more severely affected than others and much more prone to fractures. Many of the recommendations below, though useful for any child with OI, are in many cases more germane to the child with severe OI.

When multiple fractures are present at birth, splinting is recommended to ease the pain and maintain as normal a position as possible. These fractures by and large do not happen at birth but rather occur prenatally as the child moves in the womb. The splinting usually requires the involvement of the orthopaedic surgeon. In practice, splinting these children is technically difficult and in many cases, careful handling and positioning represents the best treatment of fractures in children with severe OI. Handling of infants with OI should be limited and undertaken with slow, methodical movements. Egg-crate foam mattresses or other very soft surfaces are sometimes advised for sleeping. It may not be desirable to always keep the baby on a soft surface as this can lead to occipital flattening or torticollis (wry neck) since active movement is inhibited. Avoid startling the baby since this can cause sudden movements that create fractures.

Lifting a child with OI should be done in such a manner as to minimize the risk of fracture. Maximize full body support when lifting by spreading fingers wide to provide a broad base of support. Before lifting a child with OI, plan where the child will be placed so handling is kept to a minimum. Always assure that the legs and arms are not caught in a blanket or other object as you lift, and pay particular attention to fingers and toes which can become caught in clothing as it is pulled on. Don't pull on the arms or legs, and avoid picking up the infant by pulling on one limb. It is best to lift under the head and buttocks. A foam pad or other support under the infant during lifting is sometimes recommended though holding the infant directly offers a greater degree of control.

The goal in diapering a child with OI is the same as that in any of the other activities of daily living: avoiding fractures. Even such movements as placing the child down on the changing table or picking him up can result in fractures and should be done with care. Once the child is on the table, with a flat hand, slide the clean diaper under the soiled one, unfasten the soiled diaper and gently pull it out from underneath the baby. Clean the baby and then fasten the new diaper. One trick in babies with painful fractures is to insert sanitary napkins inside the diaper, 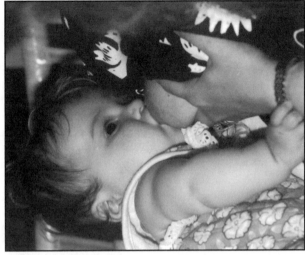 replacing them as necessary without changing the diaper. When diapering a child, care should be taken to hold the legs by the thighs rather than the ankles to prevent sudden jerking movements which could cause a break. The infant's legs should be manipulated as little as possible during the change and not bent or moved any more than necessary. Parents of children with OI should take even more precautions than other parents in preventing falls from changing tables. When dressing the baby, simple precautions can be taken to avoid fractures. The fingers are particularly vulnerable and should be protected by the care-giver's hands when pulling on shirts or outfits.

Feeding issues should also be taken into consideration in newborns with OI. Breastmilk is an excellent source of calories for virtually all young infants including those with OI, and nursing can create a special bond between mother and child. Babies with all but the most severe forms of OI should be capable of nursing, however those with very severe OI may have breathing difficulties that interfere with the ability to suck. The same care should be taken in holding and positioning the infant for nursing as for other activities. Mothers should be especially careful to avoid having the child positioned with an arm behind the back or a leg pressed against the body in such a way as to put pressure on it at an abnormal angle. After 6 months of age, an infant taking breastmilk may benefit from a vitamin supplement containing Vitamin D that is important for calcium absorption and bone formation. Supplemental calcium should be avoided in most cases since some children with OI excrete excess calcium and additional calcium intake would exacerbate the condition and could lead to kidney problems.[6] If a baby is not able to nurse or if the mother is not able to breast-feed, an option is for mother to pump breastmilk and feed it to the child in a bottle. If mother chooses to not use breastmilk, the commercial infant formulas are acceptable. Burping should be done very gently so as not to risk fractures especially of the ribs. Soft taps possibly with padding over the hand are recommended. A suggestion for picking up the child for burping is to have the baby lying on his or her back while bending over to pick the baby up. The caregiver's shoulder should just barely touch the baby at which point the infant is supported under the back and positioned on the shoulder as the caregiver moves up and backwards. Gently rubbing the back while taking gentle bouncing steps is helpful.

Baths can be a wonderful experience. Water is a protective environment for these infants, and they can float and move freely without as much risk of injury. The same precautions that apply to other children in a bathtub apply to these children. Bath rings may be helpful especially if molds to help hold the baby up can be used with them.

At the time of discharge from the hospital, a car seat will be needed. A standard car seat that reclines as much as possible that allows easy entry and exit will work best. Additional support can be provided by soft padding fitted around the baby's head. The same principles apply to strollers with those that recline and have sufficient support being preferred. The seats that do not require slipping the legs through openings will work best, especially if the baby is in a cast.

The newborn period for a child with OI need not be a traumatic time. Hopefully the suggestions outlined above will prove helpful to families and health care professionals alike in optimizing the care of newborns with Osteogenesis Imperfecta.

Note: The authors thank Dr. Michael Sussman, Chief of Staff at the Shriner's Hospital for Crippled Children, Portland Unit, for his thoughtful review of the manuscript and helpful suggestions.

Bibliography:
[1] Living with Osteogenesis Imperfecta: A Guidebook for Families. Glauser HC. (ed.) The Osteogenesis Imperfecta Foundation, Inc., Tampa, 1994.
[2] Stoltz MR, Dietrich S, Marshall GJ. Osteogenesis imperfecta. Clin Ortho Rel Res 1989;242:120-136.
[3] Binder H, Conway A, Hason S, Gerber LH, Marini J, Berry R, Weintrob J. Comprehensive rehabilitation of the child with osteogenesis imperfecta. Am J Med Genet 1993;45:265-9.
[4] Bender LH. Osteogenesis imperfecta. Orthopaedic Nursing 1991;10:23-32.
[5] The Care of a Baby and Child with Osteogenesis Imperfecta. Pamphlet Available from the Osteogenesis Imperfecta Foundation, Inc.
[6] Chines A, Peterson DJ, Schranck FW, Whyte MP. Hypercalciuria in children severely affected with osteogenesis imperfecta. J Pediatr 1991;119:51-7.

Chapter 12

Growth and Development

by Priscilla Wacaster, MD

Children with Osteogenesis Imperfecta (OI) tend to have very low muscle mass and tend be at the low end of the weight charts, if even on the standard curves. This, combined with low muscle tone, sets the children up for gross and fine motor delays, and their parents may worry about the lack of appetite and lack of weight gain. Advice about food and eating habits should contain accurate and adequate nutrition information, but must be tempered with common sense. One must avoid the temptation to encourage the parents to feed the thin child foods rich in fat and calories in order to reach unreasonable weight goals. Obesity in an adult or child with OI is not desirable, and eating habits established in childhood are very difficult to change. The information in this chapter may be used to augment the physician's common sense with facts.

Birth Data

Birth weight, length, and head circumference were studied in 127 full-term infants with OI Types I, III, and IV by Vetter, et. al.[1] The data is summarized in Table 1 and compared to standard birth data from <u>Nelson Textbook of Pediatrics</u>, 14th edition.[1,2] Unfortunately, there is no published birth data for infants with OI Type II.

Table 1

| | Type of OI | | Non-OI Standard | |
	I & IV	III	5th percentile	50th percentile
Median birth weight (gm)	3025	2540	2540	3270
Median birth length (cm)	50	44	46.4	50.5
Median birth head circumference (cm)	34.5	33	32.6	34.8

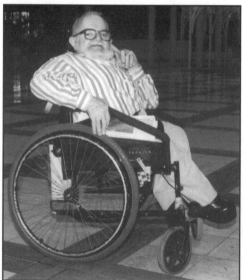

Life Expectancy

Persons with Type I OI can anticipate having an average lifespan, and several have been known to achieve ages into the 90's. Persons with Type II OI sometimes are stillborn or die shortly after delivery, while others succumb to respiratory infections or other causes of death within the first few years of life. A handful of persons with Type II OI have survived into the teen years, and one person is in his early twenties and doing well. A few persons with Type III OI die from respiratory infections in the first few years of life, but many reach adulthood and independent, self-supported living, often marrying and raising children of their own. Several persons with Type III OI have lived beyond age 60, but frequently, respiratory difficulties or other causes claim lives in middle adulthood. Persons with Type IV OI, in general, are considered to be somewhere in between Types I and III, and with regard to life expectancy, the same holds true. Persons with Type IV OI may live an average lifespan or may succumb to respiratory difficulties in middle adulthood, depending on the severity of spine and chest deformities.

Growth

There are two published growth charts for persons with OI Types I, III, and IV. The following data is taken from Vetter, et. al. and Marini, et. al. as referenced at the end of this chapter, as well as from growth data provided to the author by several individuals with OI. Persons with Type I OI typically are at a the low end of the weight charts, usually following the curve, but perhaps at the fifth percentile or lower. Height in persons with Type I OI can be average or may be slightly below the fifth percentile, but again, the pattern of growth follows the standard curves. In contrast, persons with OI Type III begin near or below the fifth percentile in weight and length then experience growth which follows the curve until 12 to 18 months of age at which time the child begins to level off with very little change in height and only gradual gains in weight. The persons with Type IV OI can also expect weight and height to be below the fifth percentiles, but growth tends to parallel the standard curves. A leveling off in weight is often seen around 18 to 24 months of age which increases the difference between the child's curve and the fifth percentile. The child usually resumes growth parallel to the standard curves in the preschool years. Head circumference is usually within normal limits for age in children with OI. But, if the child experiences an increase in head size crossing percentile lines, the child should be evaluated for hydrocephalus, which often occurs in persons with Type III OI and is seen in almost every person with Type II OI. Again, unfortunately, there is no growth data published on children with Type II OI.

The following height and weight graphs are representative examples, not standards, of how children with OI Types I, III, or IV may grow. Individuals may vary from this data as especially persons with OI Type I (as studied by Vetter, et. al. and in the author's personal experience) show a wide distribution of weight and height. Children who fall significantly below these curves should be evaluated for treatment with growth hormone. Please see chapter 13 for further details.

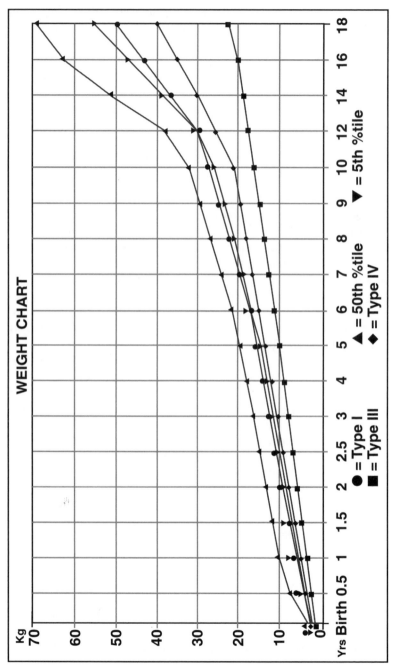

Standard (non-OI) fifth and fiftieth percentile data taken from <u>Nelson Textbook of Pediatrics</u>, 14th edition, pp. 22-23.

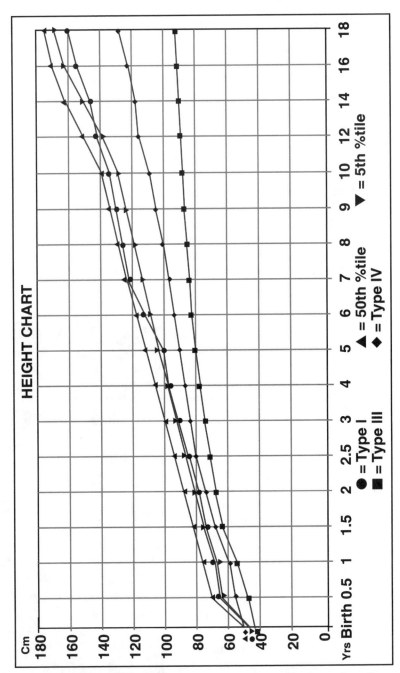

Standard (non-OI) fifth and fiftieth percentile data taken from
<u>Nelson Textbook of Pediatrics</u>, 14th edition, pp. 22-23.

Development

Cognitive development is usually normal to above normal, with advanced verbal skills. Often early intervention providers and preschool special educators are pleasantly surprised when dealing with the children with OI because the verbal skills may be two to three years ahead of the achieved age.

Fine motor skills can be mildly delayed due to hypotonia and hyper-mobile joints. Older children and adults may find writing very tiring and use computers or electric typewriters for school work. Dressing skills, such as buttoning, may be difficult to obtain, and persons may have to be selective in their choice of clothes for ease of dressing.

By age six to nine months, gross motor skills are often two to six months delayed, even when prematurity is considered. Hypotonia is usually the cause for the delay, and gross motor delay becomes more marked when the child experiences fractures. The child and family will greatly benefit from early referral to early intervention providers.[4] Physical therapists assist the child with sitting, standing, ambulation (as appropriate), and rehabilitation following fractures. The physical therapy should continue while the person is in a cast in order to maximize strength in the other limbs and trunk so that after the cast is removed, the person can rehabilitate as quickly as possible. Swim therapy is especially helpful as is recreational or competitive swimming for older children and adults.

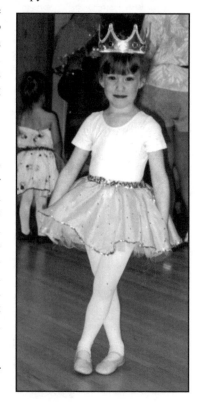

Education

Most areas of the U.S. have provisions for preschool special education for children aged two to five. Children with OI often qualify because of orthopaedic impairment and may receive physical and occupational therapy through the school for minimal or no cost to the family. The class size is generally small (six to eight children with a teacher and an assistant), and most schools attempt to place children of relatively equal cognitive skills together. Unfortunately, many school districts are quite small, and a child with OI might find himself in a room with children whose cognitive skills are much below his own. Therefore, it may be more appropriate for the child with OI to be in a regular day care setting with age appropriate peers. Many families have appreciated the assistance of their physicians in insisting that their children with OI receive the therapy needed (and maybe a personal assistant) at the school's expense while attending a private institution. "Least restrictive environment" is the term used in the federal law requiring states to provide services for children with disabilities.

Having a child with OI in the day care setting can create some unusual circumstances, and the staff of the day care center or the private individual caring for a child with OI may request that the child's physician make a site visit or speak with them regarding OI and how to appropriately handle the child. The family will also appreciate efforts made by the physicians to ease the transition into day care or preschool.

For kindergarten through twelfth grades, many children with OI attend public school with good success but some parents prefer to have their children in private school where the class size is typically smaller and the buildings less immense. Some children with OI have the benefit of an assigned aide to assist in changing classrooms or toileting following a fracture or if the child utilizes a wheelchair. Elementary school years are typically good years for children with OI. Peers tend to be accepting of the children and their limitations, including casts and wheelchairs, though some children can be treated cruelly on occasion. Junior high and high school can usher in great emotional crises of identity and self-esteem in any child, but these crises may be magnified in the child with OI especially if short stature, lack of mobility, or limb deformities are present. Academically, the children with OI tend to do very well, often graduating at the top of the class.

Many persons find confusing the difference between home schooling and home bound learning. Home bound learning consists of a public school tutor going to the home or hospital to assist the child in the completion of assignments in which the child's class is involved or, in some instances, a public school tutor preparing

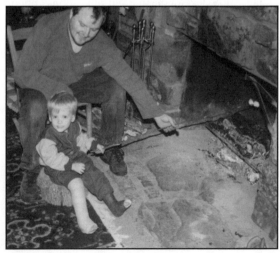

and teaching a child with a disability in the home. Many persons with OI have utilized this resource when surgery or fracture necessitates a long rehabilitation. Many adults with OI recall resentment secondary to isolation from peers and do not recommend home bound learning as a long term solution; most accept the additional risk of injury in order to have interaction with peers.

Home schooling has become a popular choice for many parents in recent years when the family has concerns about the curriculum or environment of the public school, and thousands of parents across the country are teaching children at home using a variety of available curricula. It is not surprising that many parents of children with disabilities are finding this an attractive option as well. Academically, children who are home schooled score very well on national standardized tests, and many go on to successful college

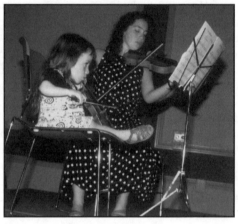

careers. The issue of peer contact is often listed as a concern for all children who are home schooled, but community resources such as houses of worship, sports teams, music or dance lessons, and scouting are available as well as neighborhood children to provide appropriate peer interactions.

In conclusion, the physician caring for a child with OI can greatly enhance the developmental and educational opportunities available to the child by early referral into early intervention, by becoming involved in the development of the plan for services for the child in special education, and by supporting the child and family in whatever educational decisions the parents make. The child with OI should have many years to benefit from the childhood experiences he or she has.

References

[1] Vetter U, et. al. Osteogenesis imperfecta: A clinical study of the first ten years of life. Calcif Tissue Int 1992;50:36-41.

[2] Behrman R, (ed.). Nelson Textbook of Pediatrics, 14th Edition. Philadelphia: W.B. Saunders Co., 1992. Page 22-23.

[3] Marini JC, et. al. Evaluation of growth hormone axis and responsiveness to growth stimulation of short children with osteogenesis imperfecta. Amer J Med Gen 1993;45:261-264.

[4] Solomon R. Pediatricians and early intervention: Everything you need to know but are too busy to ask. Infants and Young Children 1995;7(3):38-51.

13

The Case For Growth Hormone Therapy

by Donna King, PhD

The anabolic, or tissue-building properties of growth hormone (GH) have been recognized for decades. When administered to young animals and children before their growth plates have closed, growth hormone promotes bone lengthening and an ultimate increase in height. When administered to skeletally mature individuals or if overproduced in them as the result of an endocrine disorder, growth hormone promotes thickening of the bones without an increase in their length.

Is More Bone Necessarily Better Bone?

Too much of a good thing can certainly cause more problems than it solves. Acromegalics, people who produce too much growth hormone after reaching skeletal maturity, deposit additional bone at their joints, causing painful stiffening and arthritis. Excess bone deposition also changes their facial features, making them appear coarse. Furthermore, growth hormone excess can generate imbalances of other hormones, such as those affecting fertility and lactation.

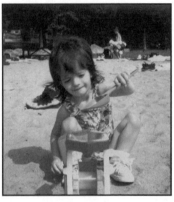

In 1985, recombinant DNA techniques allowed the development of standardized pharmaceutical preparations of human growth hormone in sufficient quantity to make them generally available at affordable prices. Genentech markets two similar formulations called Protropin® and Nutropin®. Eli Lilly markets a version of human growth hormone called Humatrope®. Recombinant human growth hormone has been approved by the Food and Drug Administration for treatment of short stature in children that have been characterized as growth hormone-deficient. Extra-label use for treating children that are not growth hormone-deficient or may not fit the clinical definition of short stature (two standard deviations or more below the mean height for chronological age, or approximately the third percentile) is not uncommon. Enhanced growth rate during the months of treatment is generally achieved in those children whose growth plates have not closed. However, it is important to note that these are primarily anecdotal observations, and very little scientific research has been conducted to document the efficacy and safety of such treatments on children who are not actually GH-deficient.

The special problem faced by patients with Osteogenesis Imperfecta (OI) is that the bone matrix is faulty. Hormonally coaxing bone cells to deposit greater quantity of the same inferior matrix will not necessarily strengthen the biomechanical performance of their bones. In the few documented cases of GH therapy for patients with OI, the treatment of each patient was individualized. This meant that few global conclusions could be drawn. In this chapter we will consider treatment of human patients with OI first, then briefly summarize some relevant research using laboratory mice.

The prospects for future treatments for OI using gene therapy are covered at the end.

Treating Patients With OI Using Recombinant Growth Hormone

It is known that children with OI have received recombinant GH treatments in the U.S. and Australia, but all have been treated on an individual basis by their physicians. The actual number of children treated is difficult to estimate, and very little has been published to date about their progress. At least ten anonymous patients with OI have been followed since 1985 in the National Cooperative Growth Study (a surveillance study of users of recombinant growth hormone products) without reports of any adverse effects of their growth hormone therapy. Two reports assessing hormone levels and growth response were published in 1993 by Dr. Joan Marini's laboratory at The National Institutes of Health and are summarized here.

Taking a conservative approach, Marini and colleagues first ran extensive tests in twenty children with OI to characterize key aspects of GH function.[1] They determined whether GH secretion was normal and whether the levels of other hormones maintained their normal relationships to GH levels in these children. Two patterns of hormone abnormalities were recognized, but none of the children fit the standard classification for GH deficiency. No correlation was found between the GH test results and the severity of OI or height of the children. The growth rate doubled for the single eleven year-old child with mild OI who was treated with recombinant GH for six months. Changes in bone strength or fracture frequency were not addressed in this pilot study.

A second publication describes two more children with OI who received recombinant GH treatment (0.1 units/kg of body weight three times per week) for at least six months.[2] Prior to treatment it was determined that these children were capable of synthesizing and releasing GH, but at somewhat less than normal levels. Their growth rates doubled during their treatment and no increase in

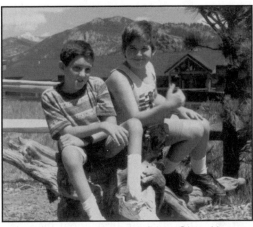

Brothers: the one on the left has OI and is two years older than the boy on the right.

fracture rate was experienced. Future publications from this group are expected to report on bone density and turnover in young patients with OI who have been treated with GH.

Is Growth Hormone Therapy an Option for My Patient?

Does the patient have short stature? Would they like to increase their growth rate and ultimate height? Are their growth plates still active, as assessed by chronological age and radiographic or scanning techniques? Growth plates close in approximately the mid-teen years, but the timing of this event is affected in each individual by gonadal (sex) hormones, nutritional status, and other factors. Closed growth plates and any evidence of a tumor are the two contraindications for recombinant growth hormone treatment.

The physician is advised not to promise stronger bones or decreased fracture frequency. If the likelihood of increased stature is proposed as the primary outcome of the therapy, then the patient and their family are not likely to be disappointed. Fracture frequency is dependent on so many variables (as examples: the specific genetic mutation, activity level of the patient, accidents, their age) that improvement in bone strength becomes a highly subjective judgment with each patient. One important question remains unanswered by researchers: If the final stature is increased, does this put additional stress on brittle bones? Ideally no adverse effects would be experienced, skeletal height would be enhanced, and the patient's quality of life would be improved. Considering the highly variable nature of OI symptoms, a large-scale clinical trial on recombinant growth hormone therapy would be required before informed judgment could be made. Ultimately, we might learn that an optimized therapy might involve a combination of growth hormone and one or more other drugs, bisphosphonates, for example.

Growth Hormone Research – Hope for the Future

For the last fifteen years scientists have been able to engineer genes and put them into mouse embryos. The mice that develop from those embryos are termed transgenic. Transgenic mice express their engineered gene and pass it along to offspring, enabling large-scale studies on how the gene performs and how it influences the mice physiologically. These mice allow scientists to run genetic engineering experiments that could not or should not be done with human volunteers. GH was one of the first genes to be investigated in transgenic mice. When the GH transgenes were expressed systemically (meaning throughout their bodies, with growth hormone released into their bloodstream) the transgenic mice grew larger than normal mice. But aside from an extended growth period and a proportional increase in bone sizes, there was little that appeared unique about the bones of these mice.[3] Continuous systemic administration of recombinant GH could be expected to produce essentially the same result in a mouse.

Several years ago a human growth hormone (hGH) transgene was engineered to be expressed specifically in osteoblasts, the bone-building cells. Transgenic mice expressing hGH right within their osteoblasts produced bones that were a little longer and stronger than normal.[4] But these researchers ultimately concluded that the transgenic bone material was actually no stronger than that of normal bone. The enhanced biomechanical properties were attributed solely to the increased size of the transgenic bones.

My laboratory has been conducting work on transgenic mice that make hGH in the red blood cell lineage of their bone marrow.[5] These mice are similar to the osteoblast-hGH transgenics just described, with one important difference: their osteoblasts respond differently to hGH that comes from neighboring marrow cells as opposed to hGH that they produce themselves. Their bones become thicker and stronger and sometimes longer than normal. When these transgenics were cross-bred to *oim* mutant mice (a line of laboratory mice that exhibits mild to severe OI symptoms), the femurs of the mildly affected mice were strengthened to the extent that their biomechanical

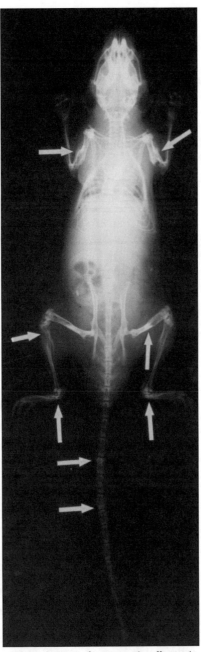

X-ray image of a severely affected nontransgenic oim *mouse indicating many recent and healed fractures.*

strength fell within the normal range. However, the bones of severely affected mice were not helped at all. While some of these results are encouraging, there are scores of unanswered questions that must be addressed before any kind of clinical therapy could be developed from this line of research. We are currently characterizing the cellular and molecular structure of the bone tissue and exploring the hormonal basis for the changes in the transgenic and *oim* mouse bone quality.

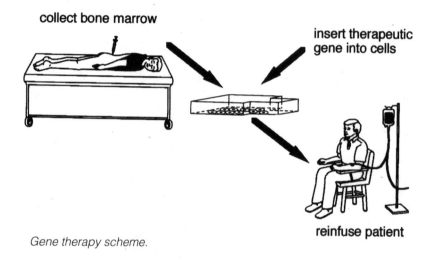

collect bone marrow

insert therapeutic gene into cells

reinfuse patient

Gene therapy scheme.

How About Gene Therapy to Treat Bone Deficiency Disorders?

More than one hundred gene therapy clinical trials are ongoing today. They are investigating gene-based treatments for health problems ranging from rare genetic disorders to cancer to AIDS. Nobody has yet proposed a gene therapy strategy for treating a bone disease, in part because bone cells are difficult to manipulate inside the human body. Scientists are currently exploring two alternative strategies in laboratory mice to get around this problem.

One possible strategy involves engineering marrow cells that are not bone precursors to simply produce extra growth factor(s), like the growth hormone transgenic mice described above. The high local concentration of growth hormone or other growth factors in the marrow might convince neighboring osteoblasts in the bone to work harder.

Another strategy exploits a special subpopulation of bone precursor cells called stromal cells that can be isolated from the bone marrow. Researchers are investigating ways to safely collect these cells from an individual, re-engineer them genetically, and return them to bone marrow cavities. From there they might be induced to mature and incorporate themselves into neighboring bone, strengthening it in the process. For patients with OI this would mean that their bone could become a mixture of cells expressing a mutated procollagen gene and some engineered to produce proper procollagen. There is some precedence to indicate that this approach could be successful. People without OI characteristics are sometimes identified as being mosaic for the OI mutation. This usually happens after the birth of their second child affected with OI, strongly implicating a parent as the source of the mutation rather than the occurrence of random mutations in the children. The relevant point is that the functional quality of mosaic bones is not necessarily compromised; they are not unusually brittle, deformed, or shortened. Achievement of the same result through gene therapy techniques may become possible in the future.

If you would like to know more about the issues discussed in this chapter, here's where to find more information:

I. Genentech is the biotechnology company that makes the growth hormone formulations Protropin® and Nutropin®. The Genentech web site offers extensive product information and recent developments.

> Genentech web site: http://www.gene.com
> Genentech, Inc.
> 60 Point San Bruno Boulevard
> South San Francisco, CA 94080-4990
> phone (415) 225-1000

II. Eli Lilly and Company is the source for the Humatrope® growth hormone formulation.

> Eli Lilly and Company
> Lilly Corporate Center
> Indianapolis, IN 46285
> phone (800) 545-5979

III. NIH web site: http:text.nlm.nih.gov

This web site connects you to the National Library of Medicine's HSTAT (Health Services/Technology Assessment Text) at the National Institutes of Health. Browse several collections of general health information or submit a key word for search.

IV. G. Ross, R. Erickson, D. Knorr, A.G. Motulsky, R. Parkman, J. Samulski, S.E. Straus, and B.R. Smith. Gene therapy in the United States: A five-year status report. Human Gene Therapy 7: 1781-1790 (September 10, 1996).

The scientific journal Human Gene Therapy is published every 20 days. It can be found in medical school libraries and libraries of many universities. In addition to scientific articles, the journal frequently publishes special features and editorials on ethical, legal, and regulatory issues concerning gene therapy. A free reprint of the above article can be obtained by contacting one of the authors: Dr. Brian R. Smith, Yale University School of Medicine, 333 Cedar Street, P.O. Box 20835, New Haven, CT 06520-8035.

Cell Therapy for OI

Another approach, being studied at St. Jude Children's Research Hospital, is allogenic bone marrow transplantation as a form of cell therapy for OI. Bone precursor cells reside within harvested bone marrow and can be transplanted in animal models. Physicians are testing the hypothesis that these bone precursor cells can be transplanted in children, will go to bone, and will contribute normal bone to the OI bone. The result will be mosaic bone, which as stated above, is functionally better than OI bone. Currently, the St. Jude Cell and Gene Therapy Program, in collaboration with investigators from around the country, is conducting a pilot study of bone marrow transplantation as treatment for children with severe OI. The hypothesis predicts that the resultant mosaic bone will reduce the severity of the symptoms, effectively altering a child's phenotype from a severe to a more moderate or mild one. More information may be obtained from or patient referrals directed to Dr. Edwin Horwitz at the address below.

Edwin M. Horwitz, MD, PhD
Division of Bone Marrow Transplantation and
　Cell and Gene Therapy Program
St. Jude Children's Research Hospital
332 N. Lauderdale
Memphis, TN 38105

References:
[1] Marini JC, Bordenick S, Heavner G, Rose S, Hintz R, Rosenfeld R, Chrousos G. The growth hormone and somatomedin axis in short children with osteogenesis imperfecta. Journal of Clinical Endocrinology and Metabolism 1993;(a)76:251-256.
[2] Marini JC, Bordenick S, Heavner G, Rose S, Chrousos G. Evaluation of growth hormone axis and responsiveness to growth stimulation of short children with osteogenesis imperfecta. American Journal of Medical Genetics 1993;(b)45:261-264.
[3] Oberbauer AM, Currier TA, Nancarrow CD, Ward KA, and Murray JD. Linear bone growth of oMT1a-oGH transgenic male mice. American Journal of Physiology 1992;262:E936-E942.
[4] Tseng KF, Bonadio JF, Stewart TA, Baker AR, Goldstein SA. Local expression of growth hormone in bone results in impaired integrity in the skeletal tissue of transgenic mice. J of Ortho Res 1996;14:598-604.
[5] King D, Saban J, Flay N, Zussman M, Havey R, Sparks S, Patwardhan A, Schneider G. Localized production of growth hormone improves bone quality in a mouse model of osteogenesis imperfecta. Journal of Bone and Mineral Research 1996;11(suppl. 1):S114.

Chapter Chapter Chapter Chapter Chapter

14

Motor Performance: Succeeding Despite Brittle Bones

by Holly Lea Cintas, PhD and Lynn H. Gerber, MD

Introduction

Children with Osteogenesis Imperfecta (OI) are individuals and their performance levels are as varied as those of nondisabled children. Given individual differences, common problems are shared by individuals with OI, particularly Types III and IV, which may be obstacles to the performance of everyday activities. The objective of this chapter is to identify obstacles to performance and interventions designed to minimize or compensate for them. The goal of rehabilitation is age-appropriate independence in physical, cognitive and social domains of function. In general, infants and children with OI bring intelligence and strong social skills to problem-solving related to performance.

Team Approach

Identifying performance priorities requires consensus among all team members, and infants and children with OI are critical players. Candid communication between parents and rehabilitation specialists fosters independence with potential for positive transfer to children. Members of the rehabilitation team include physicians, who evaluate the rehabilitation needs of children with OI, educate families, and refer to other professionals as needed. Physical therapists analyze obstacles to motor performance and teach families interventions and compensatory strategies to enhance functional motor skills. Occupational therapists correlate daily performance tasks with specialized devices to increase independence in all activities, including eating, dressing, and toileting. Orthotists fabricate braces to maintain limb alignment and improve mobility. Additional team members may include nurses, social workers, teachers, psychologists, biomechanists, and engineers.

Motor Tasks

Cross cultural studies have described varied ascent routes to walking and children select from a variety of locomotor styles based on an integration of factors. However, certain motor experiences define the progression from infancy to standing up to walk, and infants and young children with OI face obstacles peculiar to this disorder which influence this progression. Typical motor performance tasks are presented in Table 1 as a baseline for discussion of problems and interventions

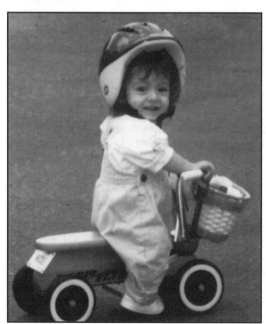

Suited up for travelin'. Age: 20 months.

specific to children with Types III and IV OI.

Splints and Braces

Orthoses, the technical term for splints and braces, serve several purposes. They may provide support for a body part, thus helping to maintain a functional position; they may immobilize a joint; they may create motion using hinges or rubber bands; they maintain alignment. There is no data, at this time, proving that they prevent deformity or fracture.

For rehabilitation of children with OI, braces are usually used to promote locomotor function. Long leg braces with a pelvic band or waist belt (HKAFO: hip knee ankle foot ortho-

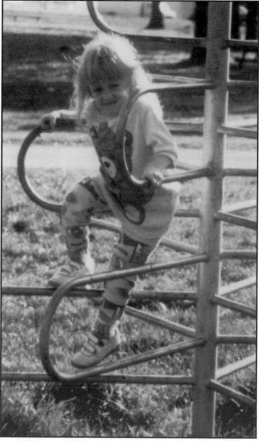

Climbing with her braces on. Age: 10 years.

ses) are designed to assist children assume the upright position by stabilizing the hip joint. Knee ankle foot orthoses (KAFO), extending to the midthigh, maintain alignment of the knee and ankle to minimize deforming forces at the knee.

Short leg braces are usually used to align and support the foot and ankle, minimizing ankle sprains and reducing abnormal walking patterns. We would like to think they help preserve bony alignment, but there have been no convincing studies to show this. Ankle foot orthoses (AFO) extend above the midcalf, provide maximal support for the ankle, and are often referred to as molded ankle foot orthoses (MAFO). Ankle and foot motion increases as brace height is reduced and soft custom support insoles represent the minimal intervention to influence foot alignment and function.

Standing is desirable for all individuals with OI to promote independence in transfers and maintain hip joint mobility. A standing frame may be

Table 1

Motor Task	Purpose	Obstacles for individual with OI	Interventions
Head up in prone leading to weightbearing on forearms (infancy)	Beginning of progression to overcome flexed position at birth; means by which infants strengthen back and leg muscles to prepare for sitting and standing	Muscle weakness and body proportionns may make this position more challenging than lying on the back; parents may be fearful of chest compression and SIDS	If infant resistant, may start with parent standing, holding infant against chest, slowly transition to parent lying flat on back; work up to infant on firmer surfaces, then infant on foam in bathtub for water work daily
Kicking in supine (infancy)	Early reciprocal kicking against gravity is means of building leg strength and gaining sense of independent movement	Weakness and frogleg position may interfere with ability to kick; babies with OI often spend too much time in supine, contributing to problems with hip flexion contractures later	Balanced positioning in prone, supine, and sidelying, to provide range of movement experiences. Daily back-lying on foam in bathtub, water level to ears, to promote playful kicking
Reaching in sidelying (infancy)	Opportunity to link hand and body movements and gateway to rolling	Bowing deformities and arm fractures	Position infant with freedom to roll slightly forward or backward and encourage this
Rolling	First form of locomotion; sequential rolling also used by children coming out of a hip spica cast	Lack of opportunity in varied body positions; head size; arm and back weakness; difficult to free bottom arm; behavioral resistance to passive, imposed exercise	Risky to impose passive rolling; respond to child's active efforts by helping to go a little further; use varied body positions to build up strength and promote satisfying increments of change

Sitting	First upright posture; position most frequently chosen by older children and adults with OI	Poor back alignment if introduced before infant has sufficient neck and back strength to support trunk; source of hip weakness and flexion contractures if sitting by children or adults is not balanced by daily standing, walking, or prone positioning	Short term use only (30 min) of infant devices which promote rounded back, alternate with prone position, or side-lying. Avoid encouraging forward propped sitting, but introduce infant sitting with erect back alignment. Avoid sling seats in wheelchairs for children and adults, choose contour or firm seats promoting level pelvis
Transfers in and out of sitting	Essential for all body transitions except rolling and scooting on buttocks	Arm weakness and fractures, or fear of fractures, are major obstacles	Early infant prone experience provides arm support practice; encourage independent efforts to transition from prone<>sitting, supine<>sitting even though it may take longer; avoid passively imposed arm support and trunk rotation interventions; custom-molded arm splints may be useful; transfer board or incline wedge may be helpful to support independent transfers for children and adults
Crawling or creeping	Interim mode of locomotion between rolling and walking. 12-13% of non-disabled children do not crawl before walking with no ill effects	Arm and hip weakness may preclude crawling, but children with OI who wish to crawl should not be discouraged	Intervention time and resources are better spent on other activities. Static positioning on hands-knees reinforces hip flexion contractures and should be avoided. Children should not be prevented from crawling up<>down steps, but safety measures are necessary to avoid falls

Table 1 (continued)

Scooting on buttocks in sitting	Means of locomotion frequently used by children and adults with OI	Arm and hip weakness and inability to get in<>out of sitting position may be contributory	May be essential for independent locomotion and is an important component of transfers for children and adults; intervention emphasis on increasing repertoire of strategies rather than trying to discourage this one
Pushing body backwards with feet while lying on back	Form of locomotion often present when child with OI cannot roll or get up into a siting position	Severe trunk, arm, and leg weakness, and head size, may preclude ability to move independently by other means	Preferable to no means of independent locomotion, but promoting alternative strategies, including early prone experience, should be pursued in infants
Standing	Erect prewalking posture in young children; very important alternative to sitting in older children and adults	Arm weakness is the primary obstacle to independent standing. Leg weakness, joint hyperflexibility and joint malalignment are also factors	Standing introduced when independent sitting is achieved, with close attention to knee and ankle alignment. Braces may range from simple in-shoe orthoses to use of a standing frame or HKAFO's (hip knee ankle foot orthoses)
Independent Locomotion	Walking represents the most typical form of locomotion, but compensated locomotion can, if necessary, fulfill the same purpose	Recent fracture, obesity, weakness, and joint contractures limit opportunities for walking. Loss of walking occurs due to arm and leg fractures, and surgery, so that even independent walkers need some type of wheeled locomotion	Consistent early intervention to promote some independent locomotion before introducing wheelchair. Individual needs govern choices of walkers, crutches and braces. Manual chairs are preferable for individuals who walk; power chairs with high-low option are best for fully compensated locomotion

Dressing, personal care	Important life skills requiring primarily hand and finger motor performance	Hand and finger performance are rarely limiting factors. Joint mobility may make overhead reaching difficult	Young children indicating desire to participate in undressing should be encouraged. Waiting for child to complete dressing task rather than parent finishing it faster is critical to development of independence
Obtaining food in the kitchen	Life skill essential to independent living	Height variations are primary obstacles	Structural accommodations in kitchen may be necessary for food accessibility; high-low powered locomotion provides access to countertops, refrigerator
Bathroom activities	Life skill essential to personal hygiene	Size of bathroom door most often reported obstacle to independence; weakness may interfere with ability to get onto toilet seat independently	If transfer skills are developed in infancy and early childhood, they are easily adapted for bathroom independence. Sturdy potty seat on floor, soft toilet seat, steps or incline wedge to get up to toilet, high-low sink and high-low power chair are among many adaptive devices available to support complete independence

used for young children prior to walking, often in conjunction with short leg braces. A supine stander or tilt table is useful for older children and adults. Braces can be applied in supine, and the device, manual or electric, provides the transition to standing.

Wheeled Mobility

Ambulation is a means of maintaining independent mobility and muscle strength, but it requires a level of fitness that may be unrealistic for some individuals to achieve. Some persons with OI may be able to ambulate for short distances, such as in the home; but may need assistance for longer journeys. Wheeled mobility, typically a wheelchair, is an effective way to provide independence for children and adults unable to walk in their communities. For the individual with good arm strength and modest distance needs, a manual chair is sufficient and relatively easy to transport. When distance needs are greater, the inconvenience of transporting a larger, heavier device may be compensated by the speed and distance it provides. A power chair with a high-low option may provide complete independence in transfers and mobility.

Sports and Recreation

Social activity and stamina building are among the highest therapeutic priorities. These can be addressed through the selection of recreational pursuits that reflect children's individual choices, with some guidelines to enhance safety. Contact sports and other high impact activities should be avoided. Children with OI can excel in water activities, starting as very young infants kicking in the bathtub and maturing with their peers in water sports, even competitive swimming. Diving carries a high degree of risk and is strongly discouraged. Mat activities, wheelchair aerobics, and T-ball with a designated runner allow participation in group activities for children at any level of ability.

Bibliography
[1] Binder H, Conway SH, Gerber LH, Marini J, Berry R, Weintrob J. Comprehensive rehabilitation of the child with osteogenesis imperfecta. American Journal of Medical Genetics. 1993;45:265-269.
[2] Gerber LH, Binder H, Weintrob J, Grange DK, Shapiro J, Fromherz W, Berry R, Conway A, Nason S, Marini J. Rehabilitation of children and infants with osteogenesis imperfecta: A program for ambulation. Clinical Orthopaedics and Related Research. 1990;251:254-262.
[3] Long T, Cintas HL. Handbook of Pediatric Physical Therapy. Baltimore, MD: Williams and Wilkins, 1995.
[4] Marini JC. Osteogenesis imperfecta: Comprehensive management. Adv Pediatrics 1988;35:391-426.

15

Dental Care for Patients With Osteogenesis Imperfecta

by Robert J. Feigal, DDS, PhD and Kurt J. King, DDS, MS

I. Introduction

People with Osteogenesis Imperfecta (OI) have a high risk of dental problems; most notably tooth structure breakdown, excessive wear of teeth, and dental decay. Prevention of these problems is possible with early and attentive dental care.

Improvements in dental science, as well as public and private action, have led to a marked decrease in dental disease in children. In spite of this progress, many children still suffer from dental decay and gingivitis. Recent epidemiological studies show strong evidence that disease patterns are skewed; with the bulk of dental decay occurring in a small percentage of the population. Unfortunately, the population with the highest prevalence of dental disease is made up of individuals with other contributing factors such as challenging medical conditions or economic difficulties. Families dealing with complex health care needs often forget the importance of preventive dental care.

Optimal health care must include a commitment to dental preventive and restorative therapy because general health is so intimately linked to the health of the mouth. This chapter outlines the main features of dental health care as it impacts the patient with Osteogenesis Imperfecta. Dental decay is the focus of the discussion. We specify preventive strategies to aid patients with Osteogenesis Imperfecta. Suggestions for optimal dental management of patients are included.

II. Dental Decay

Dental decay is a localized demineralization of tooth hard structure by the action of acids produced by mouth bacteria. For this process to become pathologic, one must grow sufficient quantities of undisturbed bacteria on surfaces of teeth and then feed those bacteria adequately and frequently. Major food substrates used by decay-causing bacteria are the carbohydrates that we eat in our normal diet. If bacteria are fed frequently enough, their demineralization or dissolving power overwhelms normal defense mechanisms resulting in dental decay. Decay, therefore, is an interrelationship among four factors: Bacteria, diet, tooth structure, and time. Given adequate supplies of bacteria and frequent feeding of those bacteria, dental decay can be an extremely rapid process, evidenced by children less than two years of age with decay severe enough to cause loss of primary teeth.

A. Prevention

Careful attention to detail can prevent all dental decay. In a patient group such as those with Osteogenesis Imperfecta, prevention is essential. Three areas of preventive action exist: Reduction in bacterial growth, reduction in bacterial nutrition, and strengthening the tooth structure. Each of these areas should be carefully described to patients and families since the essential preventive action must occur on a daily basis at home. Health professionals can aid in this preventive strategy by stimulating effective preventive home care, optimizing fluoride and antimicrobial use, and managing strategic use of antimicrobial and fluoride agents in the dental office.

1. Reduction of bacterial growth

Careful attention to effective toothbrushing and dental flossing reduces the mass of bacteria adhering to tooth structure, disrupting and disbursing microbial colonies that we call plaque. As simple as toothbrushing and dental flossing seem, they provide the basis of all other preventive action. Introduction to plaque control (toothbrushing and flossing) early in the life of

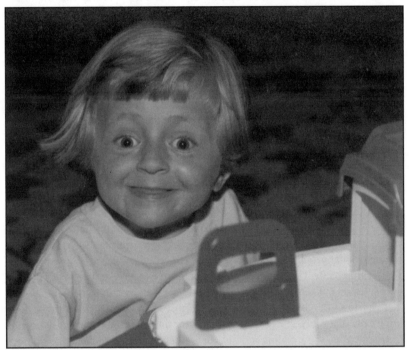

the child sets the standard for valuable life-long habits. Parents must take the lead, teaching children toothbrushing by doing it for them. Children do not possess the motor skills for effective toothbrushing until they are able to tie their shoes easily. Until that developmental milestone, parents' efforts in toothbrushing and flossing are essential. Parents should ask their dental practitioner for detailed training in plaque removal for their children. Key elements of parent involvement include a relaxed, comfortable space to work (couch, chair or bed), good lighting, positioning of the child so that the parent can see the teeth to be cleaned (head in parent's lap, etc.), and a commitment on the part of the parent to be regular with the care regardless of the child's initial cooperation.

Antimicrobial mouth rinses provide local control of bacterial growth. Some have been shown to be effective specifically against dental decay pathogens. Chlorhexidine is one of these effective agents that has become a part of preventive care for patients at times of increased risk of dental decay.

It is important that antimicrobials be used for short periods of time when prevention is to be optimized. Long term use of antimicrobials can change the normal bacteria of the mouth and also lead to staining of the teeth.

2. Reduction of bacterial nutrition

Since decay-causing bacteria produce acids and build colonies through the metabolism of fermentable carbohydrates in our own diets, it is important that prevention include attention to daily dietary intake. Fermentable carbohydrates, including sugars and short chain carbohydrates (processed starches), are the most effective foods for oral bacteria. Therefore, one must limit the intake of sugar and processed carbohydrates. In addition, the single most effective nutritional prevention strategy is minimizing frequency of intake of these foods. Less frequent eating leads to less food for the bacteria, thus minimizing acid production. On a practical basis for patients' families, this involves reducing daily snacks. We like to suggest that parents monitor snacking to include good, basic snack food at specific times of the day rather than the frequent "grazing" techniques many children are often allowed to develop.

3. Strengthening tooth structure

Optimizing fluoride intake has been recognized for fifty years as a major contributor to dental health. Fluoride incorporated into developing teeth, as well as fluoride available in the oral cavity through salivary production and locally applied agents, dramatically changes dental decay patterns. The primary effect of fluoride is to increase remineralization of very early decay lesions. Therefore, careful use of fluorides by families, patients and dental professionals is a keystone of a preventive dentistry strategy. It is important that daily intake of fluoride be optimized either through intake of fluoridated water or adding a daily supplemental fluoride tablet. In addition, topically applied fluorides can be prescribed in cases where increase preventive needs are apparent.

B. Risk Assessment

Early and effective intervention by the dentist can provide a lifetime of good oral health. Most particularly, in patients who are at high risk for dental disease or tooth deterioration, early diagnosis and planning of prevention and therapy by a dentist are extremely important. It is now accepted that the first dental appointment be scheduled at the time the child erupts the first tooth or by the first birthday, whichever comes first. This early interaction allows the dentist to counsel the family based on the individual needs of the child. The dentist can guide the family to improved habits that can optimize dental health for the entire family. Any abnormalities or early pathology can be addressed at a time before they become severe.

At each dental visit, the dentist should be making a judgment of decay risk and devising preventive strategies depending on the degree of risk. Based on multiple factors such as toothbrushing effectiveness, fluoride content of home water supply, diet habits, and past decay experience, the dentist can decide whether the child's risk is high, moderate, or low. The high and moderate risk patients should be seen more frequently by the dentist and should be encouraged to improve plaque removal and diet, optimize fluoride intake, and add topical fluoride products if appropriate. Even low risk patients with OI should be seen every six months.

Fluoride analysis and prescription

In order to accurately prescribe fluoride, a health care provider must know the fluoride content of the child's home drinking water. A water sample can be analyzed at a state or county laboratory or at most dental schools (ask your local pediatric dentist for details). Then, based on the analyzed fluoride content, a prescription can be written following the accepted dosage schedule for fluoride, recently revised in 1994 and accepted by the American Dental Association, American Academy of Pediatric Dentistry, and American Academy of Pediatrics.

Fluoride Supplementation Schedule
(mg. Fluoride ion to be Prescribed per Day)

**Fluoride Content
of Water Supply**

Age	< 0.3 ppm	0.3 - 0.6 ppm	> 0.6 ppm
6 months - 3 yrs.	0.25 mg F⁻	———	———
3 yrs. - 6 yrs.	0.50 mg F⁻	0.25 mg F⁻	———
6 yrs. - 16+ yrs.	1.00 mg F⁻	0.50 mg F⁻	———

III. Tooth Development

Commonly in patients with OI, the defect of hard tissue development that affects the bones also affects the growing teeth. Teeth start to develop in the first trimester of pregnancy, and calcification of the primary teeth starts during the second trimester. Throughout childhood and early adolescence some teeth are in active cell growth and calcification stages. The dental problem in Osteogenesis Imperfecta is primarily one of inadequate attachment of normal enamel to altered tooth dentin of the teeth. Once the dentin is exposed, the teeth wear much more quickly, and the softer dentin can be quickly attacked by decay.

About 50% of patients with Osteogenesis Imperfecta show some form of the dental abnormality usually called dentinogenesis imperfecta. The severe forms of dentinogenesis imperfecta need early and aggressive therapy to stay ahead of the tooth disintegration. All patients, severely affected or not, need attention to preventive and therapeutic dental care.

IV. Consideration of Patient Safety and Comfort

Patients with Osteogenesis Imperfecta have usually experienced multiple bone fractures and generally become anxious in the dental office. This stems not only from the dental treatment necessary but also the positioning and support necessary to protect the bones. Forces during chewing can generate a larger force than that during dental treatment, therefore, the dentist and the patient should not be reluctant to provide or have dental treatment.

The usual methods of allying apprehension that are well known and generally utilized by dentists will be most welcome to these patients. In addition, patient physical support in the dental chair will be needed. For the ambulatory patient, extra support for the neck, arms and legs should be provided. The neck support pillow that is part of most dental chairs will help protect the neck and head. Arms can be supported with arm slings or pillows and the legs with additional pillows, especially under the knees (See Figure 1). Patients who use a wheelchair because of multiple fractures and lack of mobility must be transferred to the dental chair with extreme care. The patient's caregiver can be asked to help or give direction to do this safely. Many patients have a removable custom-made insert for the wheelchair which may be transferred with the patient into the dental chair. This will provide

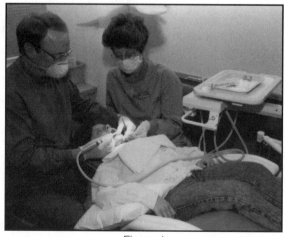

Figure 1.

maximum support and protection. Oftentimes treatment can be accomplished very well leaving the patient in the wheelchair (See Figure 2). During dental treatment great care should be taken by the operator when applying pressure such as extractions or seating a crown. Support to the head and neck region will prevent fractures when applying pressure.

Occasionally, general anesthesia is necessary to accomplish the needed dental treatment, especially for the very young patient. The same principles of support are needed in the operating room especially for the area

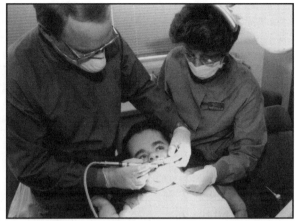

Figure 2.

of the head and neck. Manipulating the mandible and any procedures involving pressure should be done carefully with minimum pressures, and providing good support.

Planning and executing safe, comfortable dental treatment for patients with Osteogenesis Imperfecta can have a rewarding outcome for the dentist and the patient.

V. Dental Restorative Techniques

Patients with Osteogenesis Imperfecta with or without dentinogenesis imperfecta can be treated as normal dental patients with a strong emphasis on prevention. Sealants, topical and systemic fluorides, and oral hygiene all should be included. Patients with Osteogenesis Imperfecta and dentinogenesis imperfecta need early and effective hygiene treatment.

The dentinal-enamel defect on teeth with dentinogenesis imperfecta will allow rapid tooth abrasion with enamel chipping (See Figure 3). This is present in the primary teeth to a greater extent than the permanent teeth and can lead to abscesses, loss of function and decreased vertical dimension of the

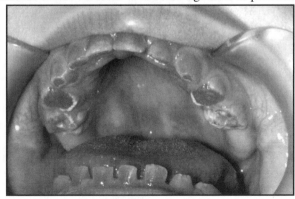

Figure 3.

jaws. The treatment of choice is to place stainless steel crowns on the molars (See Figure 4) and the newer stainless steel crowns with esthetic composite facings on the maxillary and mandibular anterior teeth. This should be done shortly after the eruption of the second primary molars. Occasionally, it is necessary to place these crowns as the teeth erupt, if the teeth are deteriorating rapidly. This seemingly aggressive treatment will provide a pleasing esthetic result, maintain vertical dimension, reduce pulp exposures and sub-

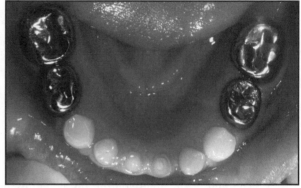

Figure 4.

sequent abscesses, and provide the patient with a functional bite.

In the mixed dentition of primary and permanent teeth (ages 6-12 years), the concerns are esthetics, comfort and preservation of tooth structure. Upon eruption of the first permanent molars and permanent incisors, an assessment of the esthetic tooth condition should be done. Usually, it is necessary to place stainless steel crowns on the first molars, however, if abrasion is not present, sealant placement followed by regular recall examinations may be adequate. The permanent incisors are often gray to blue in color and are unacceptable to the patient. The advent of bonded composites and dentin bonding agents have greatly improved the potential for esthetic restorations. All of the labial and about one third if the incisal lingual enamel should be removed, and the restoration bonded to dentin. If restoration retention depends on a bond to enamel, the restoration often will be lost as the enamel separates from the dentin.

Orthodontic treatment is not contraindicated for patients with Osteogenesis Imperfecta with or without dentinogenesis imperfecta. The same precautions for movement or pressure need to be followed. Orthodontic bands are preferred as the bonded brackets will possibly be lost or could possibly chip the enamel upon removal.

As patients enter their teens and early adulthood, esthetics, preservation of vertical dimension, function, and comfort are also important. Continued application of bonded composites for the anterior teeth or full coverage with temporary crowns will maintain the teeth. Posterior teeth may need full coverage with stainless steel crowns, onlays of cast metal, or temporary plastic crowns. Effort should be directed to preservation of the teeth to prevent enamel wear and abrasion. Adulthood allows the construction of porcelain fused to metal crowns as a more long term solution for those teeth which are prone to chipping.

Aggressive treatment from early childhood to adulthood will allow the patient to enjoy a pleasant smile, good vertical dimension, comfortable chewing, and preservation of the teeth. For patients who have not had this intervention and have lost or worn teeth, more involved treatment may be necessary. This may include bridgework, implants, or dentures.

Summary

In spite of the apparent complexities of obtaining dental care in the face of other medical needs, families with Osteogenesis Imperfecta will find quality of life improved with proper oral health. General health and comfort are optimized when the mouth is healthy. Early and aggressive attention to preventive dentistry is the key to long-term success. By using all the strategies available to families, the dental professional can offer the potential for a decay-free life.

For those with dentinogenesis imperfecta, close attention must be paid to restorative needs of the teeth. The potential for rapid tooth wear and breakdown heighten the need for establishing a relationship with a qualified dentist early in a child's life. In addition to preventive strategies, this dentist can plan necessary fillings or protective coverings for teeth in order to prevent problems from the breakdown of the affected teeth.

Many dentists are knowledgeable concerning the special needs of this population. A specialist in pediatric dentistry is most likely to have experience in the treatment of many patients with dentinogenesis imperfecta and Osteogenesis Imperfecta. With careful attention to patient comfort and support, dental treatment can be effectively delivered to patients with all levels of severity of Osteogenesis Imperfecta and dentinogenesis imperfecta.

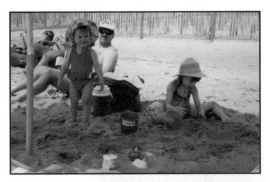

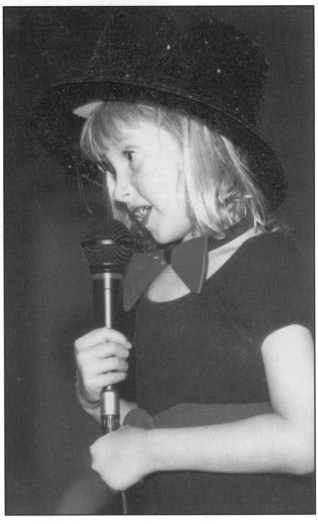

Chapter 16

The Heart

by G. Hossein Almassi, MD

Osteogenesis Imperfecta (OI) is a hereditary disorder of connective tissue affecting skeletal, ocular, auditory, integument, and dentine systems. It is a heterogeneous condition with a variety of subtypes.[1] A defect in the formation of type I collagen due to mutation within the helical regions of the alpha-1 and alpha-2 chains is believed to be responsible for this disease. The quality of the mutation and the extent of abnormal type I collagen determines the severity of the disease.[2]

The cardiovascular system is rarely involved in OI. The major structures affected are the aorta and the cardiac valves.[3] The prevalences of OI and Marfan's Syndrome are similar, yet the cardiovascular abnormalities in Marfan's Syndrome are well recognized but are infrequent in OI.[2] Cardiovascular involvement in Osteogenesis Imperfecta is similar to that seen in Marfan's Syndrome, with aortic insufficiency being the most common cardiac lesion followed by mitral insufficiency and mitral valve prolapse and, to a much lesser extent, right-sided cardiac valve insufficiencies and aortic dissection. Myxomatous degeneration of valve cusps with dilation of annulus leads to valvular insufficiency. Dilatation and enlargement of the aortic root is also seen,[4] although aneurysmal dilatation of the ascending aorta is rare. Aortic dissection was reported in two recent case reports.[5,6]

Valvular Insufficiency

Clinical Manifestations

Patients with OI with valvular insufficiency can be asymptomatic for a long period of time, but since the pathology is a progressive condition, the patient will ultimately develop symptoms.[7] In the case of aortic insufficiency, the patient usually presents with exertional dyspnea, orthopnea, and paroxysmal nocturnal dyspnea, and if left untreated, cardiomegaly and atrial fibrillation, and ultimately pulmonary edema, may develop.

In mitral valve prolapse syndrome (MVP), atypical chest pain, fatigue, dyspnea, lassitude, giddiness, and syncope may be the presenting symptoms. Progressive mitral regurgitation will develop in 15% of these patients over a ten to fifteen year period.[7] Supraventricular tachycardia and premature ventricular beats are also observed in this condition.

The major symptoms in chronic mitral regurgitation, fatigue and exhaustion, are manifestations of a low cardiac output. In severe cases, right heart failure with congestive hepatomegaly, ascites, and edema in the lower extremities are seen.

Physical Examination

The patient with aortic insufficiency characteristically will have a hyperdynamic heart with a wide pulse pressure and a water hammer pulse. A diastolic murmur is present in the left sternal border, although in patients with aortic dilatation, the murmur could be best heard on the right parasternal area. A systolic thrill may be palpable at the base of the heart or suprasternal notch.

In mitral valve prolapse syndrome, a mid-systolic click with a late crescendo systolic murmur is heard at the apex. Patients with mitral regurgitation will have a diminished S1 and wide splitting of S2. P2 may be louder than A2, and S3 may be present. Prominent systolic murmur is heard at the apex, may obscure the A2, and radiates to the axilla. This murmur is a blowing, high-pitched murmur. The cardiac impulse is usually brisk, hyperdynamic, and displaced to the left.

Laboratory Findings

In patients with advanced aortic insufficiency, the chest radiograph will show cardiomegaly with or without dilatation of the ascending aorta. Findings on electrocardiogram are left ventricular hypertrophy with left axis deviation, and the echocardiogram will establish the diagnosis of aortic insufficiency and its severity.

Patients with chronic mitral regurgitation will have cardiomegaly and left atrial enlargement on chest x-ray, which also may show Kerley-B lines. Left atrial enlargement and atrial fibrillation are the predominant findings on electrocardiogram. Electrocardiographic finding of left ventricular hypertrophy occurs in about one-third of the patients.[7] Coagulation profile and platelet count are usually within normal limits.

Management

Chronic aortic insufficiency responds well to medical therapy. Cardiac glycosides are used for atrial fibrillation and cardiomegaly. Hypertension should be treated with vasodilators to decrease the degree of regurgitation. Beta blockers, however, should be avoided.[7] Asymptomatic patients with severe aortic insufficiency and normal left ventricular function should be examined every three to six months. Serial echocardiographic examination both at rest and during exercise should be carried out. Surgical intervention is indicated in symptomatic patients with severe aortic insufficiency and impaired left ventricular function and in those with progressive deterioration of left ventricular function on serial echocardiography.

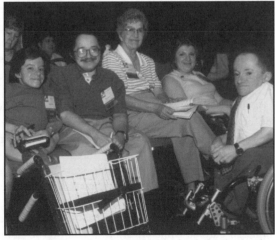

Appropriate prophylaxis for infective endocarditis is indicated in patients with aortic insufficiency as well as in all other valvular lesions.

As noted before, both aortic and mitral insufficiency are well tolerated by the patient for a prolonged period of time. The same is true for patients with mitral valve prolapse. The asymptomatic patient should be followed up every two to four years with a two dimensional echocardiogram. These patients should receive beta blockers for arrhythmias and chest discomfort. Endocarditis prophylaxis is advisable, especially in patients with a mid systolic click, late systolic murmur, and echocardiographic findings.[8] Patients with chronic mitral regurgitation will benefit from afterload reduction with an angiotensin enzyme inhibitor or oral hydralazine. This clinical improvement may last for years. Cardiac glycosides, like diuretics, are indicated in patients with chronic mitral regurgitation, cardiomegaly, and sinus rhythm, as well as in those with atrial fibrillation. Symptomatic patients, despite optimum medical therapy, and those patients with worsening cardiac function should be referred for surgical valve repair and/or replacement.

Aortic Dissection

Similar to patients with Marfan's Syndrome, patients with OI are at risk of developing aortic dissection. Patients with OI and hypertension should be placed on beta blockers to decrease the chance of aortic dissection.[12] Two recent cases of acute ascending aortic dissection have been reported in the literature.[5,6] One of these patients had had previous aortic valve replacement and both had successful outcomes following the replacement of the ascending aorta.

Surgical Therapy

Historically, open cardiac operations in patients with OI have carried a rather high mortality risk. In the majority of these cases, in patients with OI, the major underlying cause of death has been postoperative bleeding and dehiscence of suture lines. There is general belief that patients with OI have a higher tendency for postoperative bleeding, possibly secondary to some coagulation abnormalities. Platelet qualitative defects,[9] and functional defects have been blamed for this tendency. Increased platelet size,[10] defective release of platelet factor,[3] inability to aggregate normally to ADP, and elevated serum and urinary inorganic pyrophosphates[11] have all been described. Nonetheless, the clinical significance of platelet functional defects is slight.[11] An occasional patient or parent may have an increased bleeding tendency.

Patients who are deemed candidates for cardiac surgery should undergo cardiac catheterization in addition to noninvasive tests such as an echocardiogram. With better understanding of the disease itself and the availability of more sophisticated technical and technological advances along with the use of fine suture material, the operative mortality appears to be low as evidenced by the appearance of several recent reports of cardiac and aortic operations in patients with Osteogenesis Imperfecta and even in redo settings.[2,5,6,13] The operation is performed on hypothermic cardiopulmonary bypass and blood cardioplegia.

Aortic valve replacement with a mechanical valve is preferred for patients with OI who have severe aortic insufficiency and impaired left ventricular function. Aortic valve homograft and pulmonary autograft are probably contraindicated as the process of aortic annular dilatation may

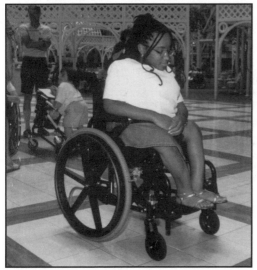

occur in these valve substitutes leading to aortic insufficiency and the need to redo the operation. Fine suture material buttressed with pledgets are used to prevent the sutures from tearing and cutting through the tissue.

Patients with mitral insufficiency are best served by mitral valve repair with any of the currently available reparative techniques. Similar to other patients with degenerative mitral valve disease, results of mitral valve repair should carry a lower operative mortality risk and better long-lasting results in patients with OI.

Aortic dissection with involvement of the ascending aorta (Stanford Type A) requires emergency replacement of the ascending aorta with prosthetic graft under deep hypothermic circulatory arrest, complimented by retrograde cerebral perfusion via the superior Vena cava for cerebral protection. If the dissection process has extended to the aortic valve, then a prosthetic valved conduit is used to replace the valve and the aortic root and reimplant the coronary arteries. My preference is to save the native aortic valve and reconstruct the aortic root with prosthetic graft material.

Summary

Cardiovascular manifestations in Osteogenesis Imperfecta are similar to those in Marfan's Syndrome but very infrequently observed. The clinical presentation and the diagnosis and treatment are similar to those of acquired valvular diseases due to other causes. There is no correlation between the severity of skeletal manifestations of the disease and the degree of cardiovascular involvement. Medical treatment is preferred for asymptomatic patients until they become symptomatic or show evidence of deteriorating left·ventricular function. The improved results of surgical therapy with valve replacement are due to a better understanding of the pathophysiology of the disease and close attention paid to the technical details during the conduct of the operation.

References
[1] Tsipouras P. Osteogenesis Imperfecta. In: McKusick's Heritable Disorders of Connective Tissue, 5th ed., Beighton P (ed.), St Louis: Mosby, 1993;281-314.

[2] Wong RS, Follis FM, Shively BK, Wernly, JA. Osteogenesis imperfecta and cardiovascular diseases. Ann Thorac Surg 1995;60:1439-43.

[3] Thiboult GE. Clinical problem-solving: The heart of the matter. N Engl J Med 1993;329(19):1406-1410.

[4] Heppner RL, Babitt HI, Bianchine JW, Warbasse JR. Aortic regurgitation and aneurysm of sinus of valsalva associated with osteogenesis imperfecta. Am J Card 1973;31:654-657.

[5] Moriyama Y, Nishida T, Toyohira H, Saigenji H, Shimokawa S, Taira A, Kuriwaki K. Acute aortic dissection in a patient with osteogenesis imperfecta. Ann Thorac Surg 1995;60:1397-9.

[6] Cusimano RJ. Repeat cardiac operation in a patient with osteogenesis imperfecta. An Thorac Surg 1996;61:1288.

[7] Braunwald E. Valvular Heart Disease. In: Heart Disease, 4th ed., Braunwald E (ed.), Philadelphia: Saunders WB 1992;1007-1077.

[8] Dajani AS, Bisno AL, Chung KJ, Durach DT, Freed M, et. al. Prevention of bacterial endocarditis. JAMA 1990;264(22):2919-22.

[9] Siegel BM, Friedman IA, Schwartz SO. Hemorrhagic disease in osteogenesis imperfecta. Study of platelet functional defect. Am J Med 1957;22:315-321.

[10] Estes JW. Platelet size and function in the heritable disorders of connective tissue. Ann Intern Med 1968;68:1237-49.

[11] Hathaway WE, Solomons CC, Ott JE. Platelet function and pyrophosphates in osteogenesis imperfecta. Blood 1972;39(4):500-509.

[12] Shores H, Berger KR, Murphy EA, Pyeritz RE. Progression of aortic dilatation and the benefit of long-term (beta)-adrenergic blockage in marfan's syndrome. N Engl J Med 1994;330:1335-45.

[13] Almassi GH, Hughes GR, Bartlett J. Combined valve replacement and coronary bypass grafting in osteogenesis imperfecta. Ann Thorac Surg 1995;60:1395-7.

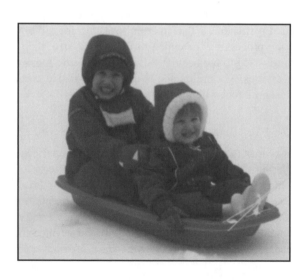

Chapter 17

The Feet

by Patrick Agnew, DPM

Disorders such as Osteogenesis Imperfecta (OI) and Ehlers-Danlos Syndrome which result in a production of inferior collagen would be expected to produce a generalized ligamentous laxity in the affected individuals. The effect of ligamentous laxity in the lower extremities has been observed to produce a variety of problems. The weakness of ligaments can result in intrauterine deformation of the lower extremities (congenital deformities). These include a higher incidence of clubfoot, medial and lateral torsion of the lower and upper legs, as well as a variety of other foot and ankle deformities. Ambulatory children may be expected to have a more flexible lower arch foot than the average population. In the affected population, a more dramatic flattening of the arch and widening and out-toeing gait are common. Pathological fractures from relatively mild or even occult trauma are common, also. Other ambulatory children with ligamentous laxity may begin to develop premature deformation of the associated structures of the foot including the toes and ankle. Deformities in this area include hallux abducto valgus (bunion), hammertoes of the flexor stabilization variety, and degenerative joint disease within the tarsus and ankle. The theoretical pathomechanical etiologies of these deformities revolves around the abnormal tension of various muscles both originating within and outside the foot.

Type I collagen is the abnormal type in Osteogenesis Imperfecta. This collagen is found in virtually all of the tissues of the human body. One might expect skin and skin structure abnormalities in affected persons such as a higher incidence of traumatic damage to the skin and nails on the feet. The damage may be occult or trivial and would be expected to result in difficult wound healing, hypertrophic scar formation, and abnormal function of the skin and nails.

Early diagnosis and recognition of the increased risk of lower extremity disease in this population is essential. Neonatal evaluation and management should include a thorough biomechanical examination. If evidence of congenital pathomechanics is encountered, it may be reasonable to attempt to correct these problems in the infant. Examples which are sometimes relegated to a more cavalier (wait and see) approach might include positional equino varus, metatarsus adductus (or varus), calcaneal valgus, and medial and lateral tibial torsion. Left uncorrected, the above abnormalities may predispose the individual with ligamentous laxity to secondary pathological compensation with the initiation of weight bearing. The treatment of these conditions is often as simple as night splinting and/or serial casting.

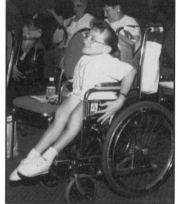

Once the child with ligamentous laxity achieves weight bearing, protection from trauma and compensatory pathomechanics is essential. Proper shoe selection should include appropriate sizing, of course. Tread designs of the shoes should be appropriate for the anticipated use. Heavy gripping tread designs may be dangerous on carpeted surfaces. Smooth slick tread designs may be equally dangerous on tile floors.

A variety of shoes may be necessary in a varied environment. Shoes should allow an effortless flexion across the metatarsophalangeal joints. Stiff shoes have been associated with an increase of traumatic falls. Shoes for this population should also provide enough room for the insertion of well designed and fitted orthotic devices. Resisting excess pronation of the subtalor joint may obviate the development of forefoot and rearfoot pathological compensation. Although long term data to verify this statement are not available, the author submits that there is little risk in the application of these devices and great risk to the patient who goes on to develop bunions, hammertoes, and degenerative joint disease in the rear foot. Studies that have condemned the use of these devices for their failure to correct the height or position of the longitudinal arch have been misguided. The shape of the arch of the foot is poorly correlated with acute disease. It is the long term pathomechanical effect of the abnormal position of the longitudinal arch that results in symptomatic foot pathology. Although orthotic devices may fail to permanently alter the shape of the arch, they may be expected to obviate these deformities through neutralizing the pathomechanical effects of excess pronation. Furthermore it may be undesirable to cause a permanent elevation of the height of the arch. The pathological effects of a very high arch have been well documented in patients with polio, Charcot-Marie Tooth disease, and others.

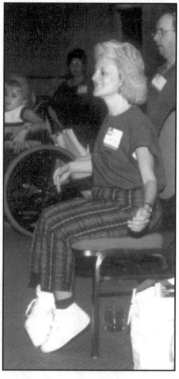

Fabrication of orthoses for this population may require sophisticated knowledge of a broad variety of designs and materials. Input from a variety of concerned specialists including orthopaedists, podiatrists, occupational therapists, and orthotists should be sought before prescribing. The orthoses should not interfere with the normal development of gait and should not irritate the skin. Orthoses should be physically comfortable and cosmetically acceptable. Orthoses should be as light as possible and provide free motion in all the normally acceptable directions.

Elective and non-elective surgical treatment of individuals with Osteogenesis Imperfecta has frequently been reported to result in a higher incidence of complications and less than satisfactory outcomes. In the author's practice, he has, however, experienced average surgical outcomes in the treatment of patients with the Ehlers-Danlos Syndrome via common and traditional podiatric surgical techniques. Meticulous dissection and hemostasis, carefully planned osteosynthesis, and intensive postoperative monitoring and rehabilitation may be expected to result in satisfactory outcomes in these individuals. Special attention to osteosynthesis is uniquely important to the population with OI. The majority of reconstructive surgery indicated in the populations with ligamentous laxity requires the cutting and repositioning of bone. These procedures might include bunion surgery, hammertoe repair, and flatfoot reconstruction. Careful weighing of the anticipated risks versus the hoped for outcomes is always essential in elective surgery. The scale is tilted further toward nonoperative therapy in persons with OI.

Once deformity has been allowed to occur and surgical treatment has been eliminated as a therapeutic option, accommodation of the deformity to

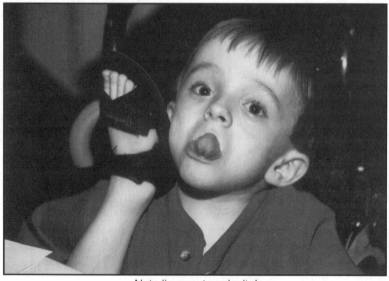

Note ligamentous laxity!

retain the best quality of life possible is the goal. This can be achieved through accommodative insoles designed to distribute weight and pressure evenly across the foot. Specialized shoes are often necessary to provide adequate room for such devices. Custom made shoes are also available. Despite their sometimes less than desirable aesthetic appearance, these are made in a variety of styles and are manufactured from extremely lightweight materials. Deformities and disease of the nails and skin may be palliated through periodic at risk debridement, padding, and accommodations by podiatric physicians. The fragility of the skin, bones, and vascular structures indicate a cautious and skilled application of this therapy. Podiatric physicians are well versed in these techniques through their experience with the elderly, patients suffering from diabetes, and persons with peripheral vascular disease.

Final Note From the Author

I once found myself in the company of a group of highly respected and nationally famous researchers in the field of connective tissue disorders. As one of the members of the medical advisors panel of the Ehlers-Danlos National Foundation, I felt embarrassed by my limited potential for altering the outcomes of our patients' disease. I was quickly soothed by the chairman of the panel who explained that although I might not be expected to discover a treatment for the genetic abnormality, the small day to day improvements in the quality of life of our patients are often greatly appreciated. I hope that the information in this chapter will be useful in stimulating further efforts to improve the everyday existence of people with connective tissue disorders.

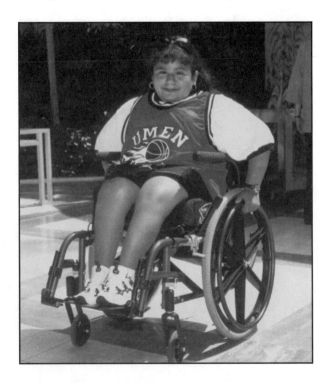

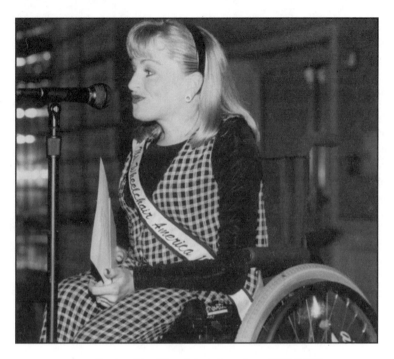

Amy Baxter, Ms. Wheelchair America, 1995-1996.

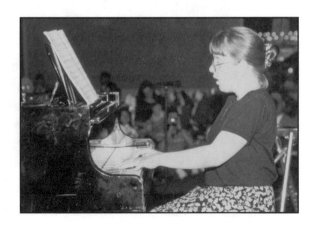

Chapter

18

Hearing
Loss

by David M. Vernick, MD

Osteogenesis Imperfecta (OI) often affects the ear leading to hearing loss, tinnitus and occasionally dizziness. Adair-Dighton first described this in 1912. Van der Hoeve and de Kleyn described the triad of blue sclerae, frequent fractures, and conductive hearing loss. This triad now bears their name – van der Hoeve-de Kleyn Syndrome. Although initial assumptions were that OI was a more severe manifestation of otosclerosis – another bone disease affecting the ear – histological examination of the bone eventually proved it to be a distinct entity. While people with OI can have concurrent otosclerosis, most do not.

Most people with OI eventually develop hearing loss. Reports have shown that up to 50% of those with OI will have hearing loss by age 50. This loss usually starts in the second and third decades of life and increases with age, though some may be affected as early as three years of age. The loss can be conductive, sensorineural or both. The etiology of this relates directly to how OI affects the bones of the ear.

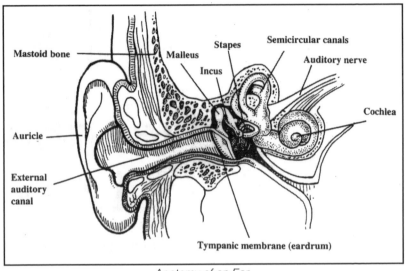

Anatomy of an Ear
(From Edwin M. Monsell, M.D., Ph.D., Division of Otology and Neurotology, Department of Otolaryngology-Head and Neck Surgery, Henry Ford Hospital, Detroit, MI. Reproduced by permission.)

Histology

The normal ear is comprised of two distinct types of bone. Enchondral bone surrounds the inner ear structures (cochlea, vestibule, and semicircular canals). Cortical bone comprises the remainder of the ear (ossicles, mastoid, petrous apex). OI can affect both of these regions.

Microscopic examination of OI bone in the ear shows a number of characteristic findings. Large remnants of cartilage are seen in the enchondral bone. Developmental delay in ossification of the enchondral bone is also seen. There is developmental delay in the formation of periosteal bone. The mastoid bone trabeculae tend to be thin and fragile. The crura of the stapes can be thin and fragile, as well. The footplate of the stapes can be thick with remnants of cartilage. The petrous apex can have a paucity of marrow spaces.

Clinically, these findings account for the easily fractured ossicles, especially the stapes crura. They also account for the marked thickening and heterogeneous composition of the stapes footplate. Both of these changes lead to the conductive hearing loss seen in OI.

Types of Hearing Loss

The middle and inner ear changes of OI lead to hearing loss usually starting in the second and third decades of life. Most often, this starts as a conductive hearing loss, due to involvement of the ossicles. The most frequently involved ossicle is the stapes. OI can cause either or both of two types of changes in the stapes. The crura or arches of the stapes can be very thin and brittle, and the footplate can be markedly thickened from immature OI bone. Fractures of the crura or immobility of the footplate can lead to the conductive hearing loss seen. The malleus and incus tend to be more fragile, as well. Fractures of all three bones have been reported.

Sensorineural hearing loss often occurs in OI. This tends to be more severe in the persons with OI Types II, III, and IV. Often the sensorineural hearing loss occurs with the conductive hearing loss, but it can occur as the only form of loss. The exact mechanisms of the loss are unclear. It has been postulated that in OI, bone around the inner ear releases enzymes that damage the vital inner ear membranes. Proof of this is lacking, however, and other genetic factors may be involved. The hearing loss usually begins in early life and is progressive. The high frequencies are involved preferentially initially. Eventually, the speech range is involved leading to marked communication difficulties.

Evaluation of Hearing Loss

Evaluation of hearing loss in patients with OI is no different than with any other patient. The evaluation should, however, begin at a much earlier age, due to the high incidence of loss seen in OI. In families with a history

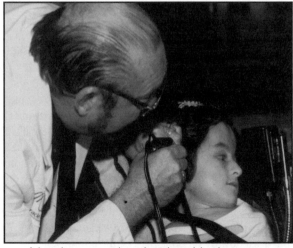

A hearing screen by a hearing aid salesperson.

of hearing loss, audiometric testing should begin in childhood by age three, In other families, a typical history is one of increasing difficulty with communication starting in the teen-age years or early 20's. Often this starts as difficulty understanding conversations in noisy surroundings. The loss then progresses to having difficulty in all conversations.

Physical examination reveals the findings of OI, such as blue sclera. Ear examinations may not show any abnormalities. Some have claimed that the ear drums look thinner. Others have reported seeing a reddish coloration to the promontory (Schwartze's sign). The significance of these observations is unclear, due to the wide variability of "normal" ears.

Hearing loss can be detected with a general office screening. Patient responses to whispered speech or quiet noises can be recorded. Tuning forks can be used to determine if the loss is conductive or sensorineural (Weber and Rinne tests). Bone conduction will be greater than air conduction in a conductive hearing loss (Rinne test). The sound will lateralize to the ear with the conductive hearing loss or away from the ear with the sensorineural hearing loss (Weber test). Once a hearing loss is suspected, audiometric testing can be performed to categorize the type of hearing loss present and quantify it. The tests involve evaluation of air conduction and bone conduction hearing levels to pure tones, testing speech reception thresholds, and speech discrimination levels. Tympanometry testing has not shown any special results in OI patients. Acoustic reflex testing can often show absence of reflexes, suggestive of fixation of the stapes. Multiple impedence test results have been reported to try to analyze ossicle and drum mobility in OI. The practical usefulness of these tests, however, in a clinical setting is unclear.

Treatment

Treatment for a hearing loss in OI involves many of the standard treatment protocols for patients with hearing loss from any other etiology – if it can be fixed, fix it, and if it can't be fixed, use amplification.

Conductive hearing loss can usually be fixed surgically if the patient wishes. The abnormal stapes bone can be replaced with an artificial prosthesis (stapedectomy). The results of this operation (Table 1) show that in three small series reported, hearing loss can be improved. The operation is more difficult than the usual stapedectomy for otosclerosis. The footplate may be much thicker and more vascular than normal, and the incus more fragile. Recent use of lasers in the operation has markedly improved the procedure. It has decreased bleeding and increased the ease of working on the stapes footplate whether it is fixed or mobile. Securing the prosthesis to the incus has been simplified, as well, with the use of a softer platinum wire prosthesis. Occasionally, the conductive loss cannot be corrected. Obliteration of the round window by OI bone may be the etiology.

Results of Stapes Surgery
in Osteogenesis Imperfecta

Table 1

	Pedersen	Garretsen	Shea
No. Of Ears	43	58	62
No. Of Patients	32	47	43
Postoperative Results			
<10dB air bone gap	62%	71%	75%
10 -20 air bone gap	21%	21%	Not reported
>20dB air bone gap	17%	8%	Not reported

If the patient has sensorineural hearing loss, or does not wish surgery for the conductive hearing loss, hearing aids are the treatment of choice. Many new advances have been forthcoming making them a better option than in the past. Miniaturization has allowed some to be placed entirely within the ear canal. Not only does this result in cosmetic improvement, but it also eliminates much of the "dead" air space between the aid and the ear drum. This allows for better quality sound transmission with less feedback at a lower level of amplification. Sound quality and flexibility of fitting hearing aids has also been greatly enhanced by the new pro-grammable dig-ital hearing aids. Fitting of the aids can be more precise as the sound spec-trum is broken down into multiple bands which can be adjusted independently. Also, the sound quality is greatly enhanced with digital processing instead of the standard analog processing used in conventional hearing

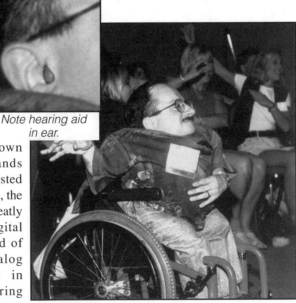

Note hearing aid in ear.

aids. Although hearing aids are far from perfect, they can benefit almost everyone with a hearing loss.

Tinnitus

Some patients with OI can hear noises in their ears even when no one else can. This phenomenon is called tinnitus. It is present in 17% of the general population and is present in up to 75% of those with OI who have hearing loss. The sound can be almost anything from a buzz to a ring to a whistle. It can be constant or intermittent. Evaluation for tinnitus involves the evaluation for hearing loss and the standard work-up for anyone with tinnitus. Treatment is the same as that for tinnitus of any other etiology, as well. If the underlying problem can be fixed, the noise may resolve. If not, then the tinnitus may be permanent.

Vertigo

People with OI can have dizziness for the same reasons as any other person. Although it makes sense that if OI can alter the inner ear hearing, it can also alter the inner ear balance system, little documentation is available for this. Future studies will hopefully clarify this picture. At present, treatment for balance disorders in OI involve the same treatment protocols as dizziness from any other etiology.

Bibliography
[1] Schuknecht H. Pathology of the ear. Philadelphia: Lea & Febiger 2nd edition, 1993;391-392.
[2] Garretsen T, Cremers W. Ear surgery in osteogenesis imperfecta. Arch Otolaryngol Head & Neck Surg 1990;116:317-323.
[3] Pederson U, Elbrond O. Stapedectomy in osteogenesis imperfecta. Otorhinolaryngol Relat Spec 1983;45:330-337.
[4] Shea JJ, Postma DS. Findings and long term surgical results in hearing loss of osteogenesis imperfecta. Arch Otolaryngol 1982;108:467-470.
[5] van der Hoeve J, deKleyn A. Blauwe sclera, broosheid van het beerwstelsel en gehoorstoornissen. Neo Tijdschr Geneesko 1917;61:1003-1010.
[6] Bergstrom LV. Fragile bones and fragile ears. Clinical Orthopedics and Related Research 1981;159: 58-63.
[7] Flintoff WM, Karmody C, Rabuzzi D. Osteogenesis imperfecta of the stapes on histological study. J Otolaryngol 1976;5(1):37-41.
[8] Pedersen U. Hearing loss in patients with osteogenesis imperfecta. Scand Audiol 1984;13:67-74.

Chapter 19

Arthritis and Osteogenesis Imperfecta

by Roger W. Lidman, MD

Introduction

Osteogenesis Imperfecta (OI) is an inherited disorder of connective tissue in which the pathogenesis appears to involve an abnormality in the synthesis or structure of type I collagen. Type I collagen is the major protein in bone matrix; thus the cardinal feature of OI is osteopenia/osteoporosis with increased susceptibility to fracture. Recurrent fractures may lead to skeletal deformity, which places abnormal biomechanical stresses on the articular cartilage of the contiguous joints. This may then lead to accelerated deterioration of that cartilage and secondary compensatory bone changes. Type I collagen is also found in ligaments, which are supporting structures of the joints. Defective support may promote hypermobility, again with excessive mechanical stress on the cartilage, leading to deterioration and degeneration. In both situations, osteoarthritic changes develop, and osteoarthritis may be a common problem for ambulatory adults with skeletal deformity or joint hypermobility.

Joint Physiology and Function

Understanding the development of osteoarthritis (OA) requires a basic appreciation of the joint both anatomically and physiologically. Amphiarthrodial joints such as the symphysis pubis and sacroilic joints are composed of flexible fibrocartilage and allow only minor rotary motion; diathrodial joints such as the knee, wrist, etc., are lined by synovial tissue, have bony surfaces covered by articular cartilage, and allow motion in all planes. The supporting elements of muscle, tendon, and ligament bring bone and cartilage into alignment to permit low friction motion – flexion, extension, and rotation of the joint – and achieve low friction load bearing.

Articular cartilage is 70-80% water by weight, but type II collagen makes up 50-60% of its dry weight; the rest is comprised of carbohydrate-protein-hyaluronic acid complexes (proteoglycans). The articular tissue, which is involved in joint motion, is separated from its surrounding elements by a capsule which is composed of type I collagen. The capsule serves to prevent hypermobility which would place abnormal shearing forces on the articular cartilage.

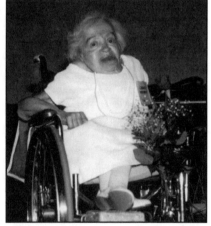

Both amphiarthrodial and diarthrodial joints preserve alignments and distribute loads in addition to permitting skeletal motion. These loads occur in everyday activities, e.g., ambulation, and may represent many multiples of body weight on a given joint. For example, with each step taken, an individual places four times his or her body weight on the hip, knee, ankles and small joints of the feet. Loading energy is taken up by muscles and tendons that cross the joint; that which is not absorbed by these surrounding structures impacts articular cartilage and subchondral bone. Therefore disruption of normal joint mechanics by ligament laxity (hypermobility) as may occur in Type I OI or by structural deformity of the contiguous bone as may occur in Type III or IV OI, may cause damage to the cartilage/subchondral bone complex.

Pathophysiology of OA

The articular cartilage is a meshwork of collagen filters arranged both parallel (superficial) and perpendicular (deep) to the articular surface. Proteoglycan molecules are arranged throughout and because of their hydrophylic nature, help to maintain the water content of the cartilage. When the collagen network is damaged, there is an initial increase in the water content of the cartilage and there is an increased net synthesis of proteoglycan. Chondrocytes, the cells involved in cartilage production, increase their activity in an attempt at repair, but their new products have inferior mechanical properties. Eventually, the cartilage softens, and vertical clefts appear (fibrillation). Fibrillated cartilage is lost into the joint space, causing low-grade inflammation and exposing subchondral bone. The bone is less successful at absorbing load and develops microfractures through its trabecular structure, which may coalesce to form cysts. In an attempt to compensate for cartilage loss there is new bone growth forming osteophytes, or spurs. Ordinarily, deformation of subchondral bone serves as a major shock absorbing structure. However, the microfractures caused by increased stress on the subchondral bone heal with stiffer, less deformable trabeculae. Stresses are then concentrated on a smaller articular cartilage surface, the cartilage fails, more stress is placed on subchondral bone, and the process accelerates.

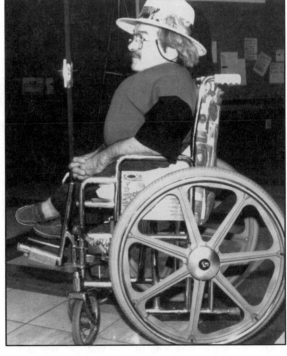

Eventually, there is bone-on-bone, thickening of the joint capsule, muscle atrophy, and chronic synovial inflammation (end-stage OA).

Clinical Features of Osteoarthritis

The most prominent feature of osteoarthritis is pain, though it is usually not present at rest, except in advanced cases. Physical activity with concomitant stress on the joint aggravates the discomfort which may be described as a dull ache or sharp, stabbing sensation, and rest usually relieves it. Stiffness with inactivity, such as after prolonged sitting, is a frequent complaint. Morning stiffness upon first arising may occur, but is generally of shorter duration than that seen in inflammatory arthritides such as rheumatoid disease. One must recognize that hip pain may localize to the groin, but could radiate to the anterior thigh or knee; radiation to the lateral thigh may simulate trochanteric bursitis. Knee pain from osteoarthritic involvement is usually localized, but may radiate distally, and inframedial radiation may mimic anserine bursitis.

The cardinal physical findings are pain with motion and possible limitation of motion of the involved joint. Crepitus, or the palpable or audible sensation of "bone against bone" may be present. Effusions may occur, but significant warmth or redness suggest a more inflammatory etiology.

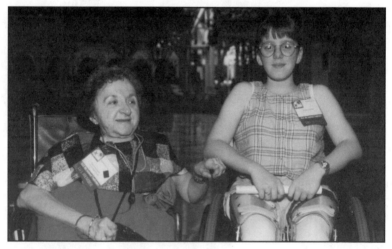

The radiographic hallmarks of osteoarthritis include joint space narrowing (reflecting loss of articular cartilage), osteophyte formation, and subchondral cysts; the latter two generally reflect advanced disease. There is usually some bony sclerosis, or increased bone density, though patients with Types III and IV may not demonstrate this; the changes of OA would be superimposed upon those of OI.

Management of OA in OI

Management goals for OI patients who have developed OA are to control pain and other symptoms and to minimize disability. Treatment

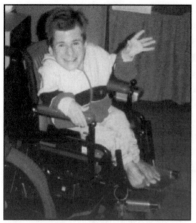

should be individualized and physicians should consider any co-existing medical problems such as peptic ulcer disease or hypertension that might influence specific drug therapy. They should also address the structural deformities from fracture disease that may require attention from physical and occupational therapy.

Non-pharmacological Therapy

Patient education, and where appropriate, education of the patient's family and caregivers is an important part of the treatment plan. Patients should be encouraged to participate in self-management programs such as the Arthritic Self-Help Course, as studies have shown significant improvement in quality of life for these who do. One may contact the local Arthritis Foundation for dates, times, and locations of the course. For those with significant impairment of their ability to perform activities of daily living (ADL), the assistance of both physical and occupational therapists may be invaluable, both for the provision of assistance devices and for instruction in exercises to maintain or improve range of motion and muscle strength. Patients with OA of the hip may benefit from orthoses to correct biomechanical abnormalities from leg length abnormalities, etc. Occupational therapists teach principles of joint protection and energy conservation.

Pharmacologic Therapy

Pain relief is the major indication for drug therapy in patients with OA as there are as yet no drugs that reverse the structural or biomechanical defects of OA. As general rule the safest drugs are the drugs of choice. Until now, nonsteroidal anti-inflammatory drugs (NSAIDS) were recommended as initial therapy, but because of recent concerns about possible harmful effects on cartilage metabolism, the minor role of synovial inflammation in the natural course of OA, and the risk of toxicity from NSAIDS, their central focus in therapy has been questioned. Although no formal studies have yet been published, a survey of community-based rheumatologists showed greater use of non-narcotic simple analgesics, i.e., acetaminophen. Doses as high as four grams per day may be used and indeed have been shown to be as effective as NSAIDS in OA of the knee. Reports of liver toxicity are generally associated with excessive concomitant alcohol intake. Renal toxicity with long-term use may be a concern, as with NSAIDS.

Toxicity remains the major reason for not using NSAIDS as first-line treatment for OA. Even "relatively young" patients on NSAIDS are at high risk for gastric bleeding, as well as possible renal toxicity. When necessary (see below), the risk of gastrointestinal toxicity may be minimized by using single preparations at the lowest effective dose, which for analgesic effect may be considerably less than the anti-inflammatory dose.

NSAIDS for analgesia may bridge the gap for those patients whose pain is unresponsive to acetaminophen and for whom narcotics, such as propoxyphene, codeine, hydrocodone, or oxycodone should be avoided for long-term use. With regard to analgesic effect, most NSAIDS are equal in efficacy. Many are now available without prescription – ibuprofen, naproxen, ketoprofen – and choice is commonly based on frequency of dosage and cost considerations. Two special considerations would be nonacetylated salicylates, such as Disalcid,™ which are associated with the least risk of renal and

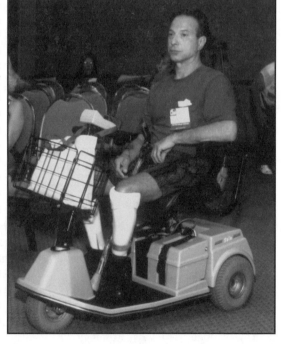

hemostatic toxicity, and indomethacin, which, because of its possible association with accelerated joint destruction in OA of the hip, is best avoided for long-term use. Furthermore, the toxicities of indomethacin – CNS, GI, renal, ocular – argue against its use as an analgesic. Finally, because of the variability in pain levels and duration in patients with OA, the use of short half-life agents, for example, ibuprofen, on an "as needed" basis is recommended.

As previously mentioned, some osteoarthritic involvement has an inflammatory component with joint effusion, warmth, etc. Such cases may require higher NSAID doses, with greater concern for toxicity, or intermittent joint aspiration. Injection of depot corticosteroids under sterile technique is then appropriate if there is no evidence of infection, but such therapy should not be performed more frequently than three to four times in a given year. There is concern that more frequent injection therapy may produce progressive cartilage damage, and patients who require more injections to control symptoms would be candidates for surgical therapy.

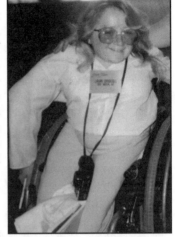

Topical Therapy

A recent advance in the symptomatic management of OA is the use of capsaicin cream, a compound that when applied three to four times a day depletes nerve endings of a chemical involved in pain transmission. Various non-prescription formulations are now available and when used as specified, are usually effective and well tolerated. Use in the groin area (for painful OA of the hip) is generally not recommended because of transient burning sensation it may produce in skin and adjacent membranes.

Conclusion

Osteoarthritis, especially of the weight bearing joints of the lower extremities is yet another complication for those patients with OI Types I, III, and IV. While there are special management considerations, most individuals are managed with the same principles as are patients with arthritis who do not have OI. Understanding of the pathophysiology of the arthritic process argues for an emphasis on pain control with the least toxic pharmacologic agents, improved function with physical and occupational therapy, and the use of self-management techniques that allow the individual to be the master, not the victim, of the disease.

Bibliography
[1] Whyte M. Osteogenesis Imperfecta. In: <u>Primer on the Metabolic Bone Diseases and Disorders of Mineral Metabolism</u>. Favus M (ed.), Philadelphia: Lippincott-Raven, 1993.
[2] Mankin HJ, Brandt KD. Pathogenesis of Osteoarthritis. In: <u>Textbook of Rheumatology</u>. Kelley WN, Harris ED, Jr., Ruddy S, Sledge CB. Philadelphia: Saunders, 1993.
[3] Hochberg MC, et. al. Guidelines for the medical management of osteoarthritis: Parts I and II. Arthritis Rheum 1995;38:1535-1546.
[4] Lorig K, et. al. Outcomes of self-help education for patients with arthritis. Arthritis Rheum 1985;28:680-685.
[5] Batcehlor EE, Paulus HE. Principles of Drug Therapy. In: <u>Osteoarthritis Diagnosis and Medical/Surgical Management</u>. Moskowitz RW, Howell DS, Goldberg VM, Mankin HJ (eds.), Philadelphia: Saunders, 1992.

[6]   Sandler AN, et. al., Analgesic use and chronic renal disease. N Engl J Med 1989;320:1238-1243.

[7]   Rashad, et. al. Effect of non-streoidal anti-inflammatory drugs on the course of osteoarthritis. Lancet 1989;2:519-522.

[8]   Brandt KD. Should osteoarthritis be treated with non-steroidal anti-inflammatory drugs? Rheum Dis Clin North Am 1993;19:697-712.

[9]   Bradley JD, et. al. Comparison of an anti-inflammatory dose of ibuprofen, an analgesic dose of ibuprofen, and acetaminophen in the treatment of patients with osteoarthritis of the knee. N Engl J Med 1991;325:87-91.

[10] Williams, et. al. Comparison of naproxen and acetaminophen in a two year study of treatment of osteoarthritis of the knee. Arthritis Rheum 1993;36:1196-1256.

[11] Deal, et. al. Treatment of arthritis with topical aapsaicin: A double-blind trial. Clin Ther 1991;13:383-395.

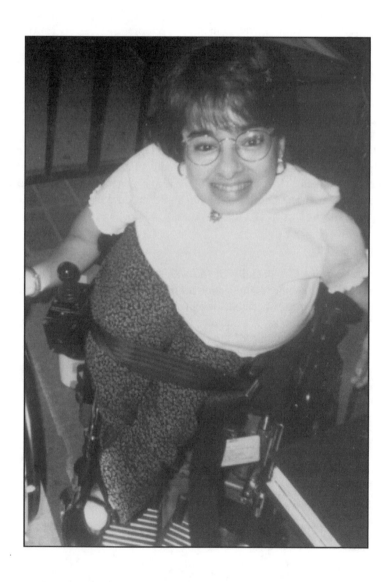

Chapter 20

Walking the Tightrope:

Juggling the Psychological Needs of the Whole Family

by Kay Harris Kriegsman, PhD

Several years ago, during a workshop for parents to deal with the feelings surrounding the birth of a child with a disability, one father submitted that the only word that came to mind when the doctor first told him his baby was severely disabled was "Broccoli".

Broccoli?

"Yes. The doctor said he would be a vegetable and all I could think of was broccoli."

Later during the conference, this father brought over his son, a handsome, crew-cut blonde teen who happened to use a wheelchair.

"I wanted you to meet Broccoli." Father and son laughed uproariously.

Obviously this father had moved through the process which allowed him to come to terms with his son's disability, which was neither to ignore the disability nor to "halo" it. He had put it into the proper perspective.

For the family with a member who has Osteogenesis Imperfecta (OI), this perspective, balancing the reality of the disability and the rest of life, is essential. Because of the on-going concern for and reality of recurrent bone breaks and other medical complications, families need added psychological resiliency to maintain equilibrium.

This chapter highlights some of the psychological ramifications of having OI in the family. It will discuss how families may maintain their buoyancy including: dealing with initial and subsequent feelings about having to live with OI; focusing on the abilities of the member with OI to attain life goals; and balancing the needs of all members of the family to maintain psychological health.

Initial Grieving Process

Becoming a parent is a challenge. Having the added dimension of Osteogenesis Imperfecta is a double whammy. Parents have to face not only the "new baby" concerns but also the physical, medical, and financial concerns relating to disability. Most parents, although not all, need to deal with their feelings about having a child with a disability in order to move on to the raising of the child without the complication of negative feelings about the child's disability or about the parent himself. Varying across a wide range, emotional reactions seen as abnormal in other situations are quite normal in this unexpected situation.

Although there are several mourning models, Schneider's 1983 (Schneider, J. The Nature of Loss, the Nature of Grief: A Comprehensive Model for Facilitation and Understanding. Baltimore: University Park Press, 1983) model is a growth model which helps people to identify, express, and validate their feelings. Presented here is the basic model with this author's additions and interpretations. This is a model based on the experiences of normal, healthy people leading to resolution.

Stage 1: Becoming aware

Parents' initial awareness is marked by feelings of shock, loss of balance, and an increased vulnerability to infection. Parents of children with

OI have identified additional initial feelings including:
> Guilt
> Anger
> Confusion
> Why me, God?
> Fear of the unknown and the future
> Fear of being different from other families
> Fear of others' perceptions
> Concern about decline in quality of life
> Concern for doctor competence and knowledge about OI
> Loneliness - feeling all alone
> Feeling distanced from others

Guilt is the feeling parents of children with disabilities most often express, but it has added meaning when the disability is a genetic condition. "Passing down" the condition or inherited tendency is a major consideration for parents with OI. Many people who have OI make an informed decision about the chances of having a child with the same disability. For them, there is a range of emotional reactions, from complete acceptance to dealing with all of the feelings presented above. Just because a parent has OI, one need not assume that he or she will by-pass the mourning.

Some children are not diagnosed until they have experienced several breaks. For these parents, the diagnosis is an answer and brings relief. Other parents, unaware of the OI, go through the trauma of being accused of child abuse. In a recent literature search, most of the articles in a medical data base concerned differentiating OI breaks from child abuse trauma. If parents have been accused of child abuse, having a diagnosis brings vindication; however, it still brings a need to deal with feelings about the disability.

Stage 2: Attempts to deal with sense of loss

Initial development of strategies to overcome the loss is the second step. The difficulty in adopting a strategy at this time is that the extent of the baby's disability is not yet accurately diagnosed. Parents at this point may feel the need to completely deny the disability or may need to see the disability as completely identifying the child. Having conflicting emotions about the baby at this time is normal.

Parents also often wonder at this stage how to describe to their extended families what is going on. It is important to urge them to reserve their energies for themselves and their child/children; if, however, they have excess energy, then they may extend themselves to others. During this time families may be supportive and comforting like a lovely blue spruce or they can be needy and nettlesome like poison oak. Some can be sources of information, respite, grounding, and support. Others are so caught up in their own grief that they become drains on the parents. Parents need reassurance that it is "okay", and sometimes even necessary, to distance themselves from such family or friends for a time while they are dealing with their management of the child and their own emotional needs.

Stage 3: Full awareness

This stage brings full awareness of the reality of the disability and its implications. Parents describe having lonely, resentful, angry, or sad feelings. They also talk about being overwhelmed by the implications of OI. Decisions are difficult to make. They display exhaustion, sometimes physically neglect themselves, and show lowered resistance to infection.

Stage 4: Time as healer

Time passes and becomes a healer. Parents learn routines, see their children survive and begin to thrive. As they begin to see that they are able to manage, their confidence begins to build. They begin to have the energy to more effectively deal with their baby and his disability needs. They report a sense of healing and an ability to deal with the loss.

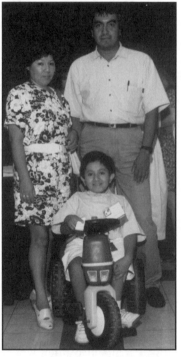

Stage 5: Resolution

Resolution and reformations take place. Parents begin to "reframe" their baby, to see their child as a person, with "disability" being a descriptor not a definer. Outwardly this movement is seen as Mom and Dad begin to rejoin outside activities and to take control of their lives.

Stage 6: Transcending loss

The last stage goes beyond disability, to transcending the loss. At this stage, parents feel balanced and achieve some serenity. They see their child as "Michael who can be winsome and bratty and demanding and bright and, oh, yes, he does use a wheelchair." The wheelchair is an integral part of his life but it does not define him.

This grief and loss model helps to resolve the gap that exists between the dream of that perfect child and the child who is. It helps re-orient parents as they pass through the disequilibrium, readjustment, reorientation and finally reframing stages.

Beyond the Initial Diagnosis

The steps above are those often experienced by parents coming to terms with the initial diagnosis of OI. Four points need to be emphasized.

1. Not all parents will need to move through these steps.

2. Not all parents will proceed through the steps in sequence. Some may skip steps or may double back to retrace steps already taken. There are also differences between the sexes or between the primary caregiver and the parent who works outside the home. In a recent OI workshop, mothers and fathers identified different mourning processes and coping mechanisms. Mothers who did the major caregiving for the child, said they had a difficult time "stopping the tears" and felt frustrated. Fathers stated that they "shelved" their feelings during work hours or when they were on the golf course. They felt they had a slower healing process, but one father added, "We feel pain. We just express it differently."

3. Parents may go through this process of grieving at other times in the child's life. For more about other periods of feeling loss, see below.

4. Extent of disability does not dictate level of mourning or need to adjust. It does present different needs and issues. The person with OI which is not observable has an identity choice: "Do I 'pass' as nondisabled? At what cost?" They often find themselves needing to explain, justify, or ask that their needs be met from skeptical teachers, bosses, or acquaintances.

What Are the Signs of a Parent in Trouble?

Differentiating the normal grieving process from clinical depression or other psychiatric disorders can be challenging. One signal that a parent is in trouble is that he seems "stuck" in a certain stage — anger, guilt, anxiety — without being able to "move on" for an excessive length of time. He may lose interest in normal life activities or dwell on his child's disability and lose sight of the rest of the family.

There are also parents who completely deny the disability and have unrealistic expectations. Others cannot move past the sense of guilt and personal responsibility for the child's condition. The trick is to differentiate between the mourning process presented above, which may be perfectly appropriate and expected, from those feelings which require professional support.

There are two levels of assistance. The first approach is to put these parents in touch with other parents of children with OI. The Osteogenesis Imperfecta Foundation (OIF) would be happy to connect knowledgeable, experienced parents with newly diagnosed families.

The second level is to suggest professional assistance. How do you suggest professional assistance? Let parents know that they are going through a difficult process which is hard for most people. Knowing that they are not abnormal, alone, or strange is reassuring. It is also helpful to be aware that there are identifiable steps (e.g. above) to this process and that one does come out on the other side. This offers hope.

Where Do You Find Professional Support?

Professional support can be located by reports of friends who have been satisfied working with a particular clinician. The OIF may be aware of therapists in some locales through their local affiliates. If, however, this route is not fruitful, there are national associations which will aid in the search.

For licensed, professional psychologists, call 1-800-374-2723 to get the phone number for each state's organization; each state has a listing of clinicians for referrals. (The Association's URL is: http://www.apa.org.) The National Registry of Psychologists has a more selective listing and may be reached at 1-202-783-7663. Branch offices of the American Psychiatric Association may be located by calling 1-202-682-6000. (The Association's URL is: http://www.psych.org/public_info/INDEX~1.HTM.)

The National Board for Certified Counselors has referral bases at 1-910-547-0607; this board certifies mental health, addictions, gerontological, school, career, and generic counselors. (The Board's URL is: http://www.NBCC.ORG.) The Commission on Rehabilitation Counselor Certification can recommend rehabilitation counselors and addictions counselors at 1-708-394-2104. To locate a social worker, call their Clinical Register at 1-800-638-8799; ask for Membership Services and then request a referral from the Clinical Register.

Prior to calling any of the referral sources, it would be wise to determine what qualities or qualifications in a therapist are desired. Sex, age, experience with disability or OI in particular, or type of therapy practiced are a few of the qualifiers clients often raise. Parents should feel completely free to ask questions so that they have the right "fit" with the professionals with whom they will work so intimately.

Dealing With the Disability Issue as the Child Grows Older.

Will you hear parents going through similar stages again? As indicated before, the answer is often yes. At important developmental stages, parents may experience this feeling of loss and hurt for their children. This is often noted in adolescence when teenagers are normally becoming social, beginning to date, or getting their drivers' licenses. Being shorter in stature, using orthopedic appliances, often being encased in a cast, or having different features will be most pronounced and hurtful during the turbulent teen years.

Another problematic developmental stage is the transition from high school to college or the work world. A challenging time for any family, it has added concerns when a young adult has OI. It is even more difficult when the person is not completely independent. Balancing parental concerns and young adult desires for autonomy creates tension within the family. An "outsider" is very helpful to sort out fears from realities at this time.

What Are the Signs of a Child in Trouble?

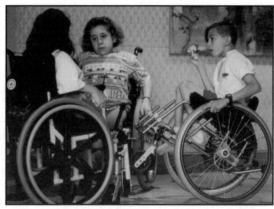

Sudden changes in behavior or in normal personality patterns are key indicators. Any child who is at an extreme – the "perfect" child or the "perfectly horrid" child – is at risk. Another possible indicator is the child who matures too quickly, at ease with adults but not his peers, or looks with disdain on the activities which are central to adolescent development.

Moodiness, depression, anxiety, aggression, eating disorders, and self destructive tendencies need to be monitored. School counselors and psychologists are often helpful as are the same cast of helping professionals suggested above.

Sibling Stuff

What is often overlooked in the family where a child has OI is the neediness of the brother or sister without a disability. During times of crisis (e.g. an OI fracture), able-bodied brothers and sisters often take a back seat and say they feel that they are ignored or not as highly valued. The ways families react reflect their individual structures and vary widely. Siblings indicate, however, that a significant proportion of the brothers and sisters feel neglected, some even wishing that they had OI so that they would receive equal attention.

Those who complain about being "left out" talk of the extra burdens they carry in terms of compensating in taking care of chores or actually caring for their sibling with OI. Their needs, they say, are not tended to so immediately or with as much concern as their sibs' with OI complaints.

Others report that parents have told them that they are "lucky" that they didn't have OI and to stop complaining. Parents may also refer to the child with OI as "special". Sibs wonder if they lack "specialness" simply because they don't have OI. Others feel that discipline is not meted out equally.

Other brothers and sisters feel that they are included and valued and feel no jealousy of the sibling with OI. They report that their parents have been careful to pay attention to their "hurts" and needs.

In a small sample, birth order in the family contributed in some measure to the way the siblings felt, with older siblings of brothers and sisters with OI reporting more dissatisfaction. This may be a normal older/younger sibling reaction or OI may impact. There is a need for research in this area.

Parents need to be encouraged to reserve energy to deal with the needs of all their children on an equal basis. They need to weigh the complaints of sibs through the "normal" calibrator of the usual brother-sister interactions. Most sibs at one time or another feel they are short-changed in parents' attentions. So it is important for parents to sift out what is normal and what is due to the impact of disability in the family. Although in times of crisis this equalization of all siblings' needs may not be possible, in times of equilibrium this is achievable.

How Parents Can Promote Their Child's Journey Toward Adulthood

Preparing any child for adulthood is no easy task for a parent. Preparing a child with a disability requires greater thought and foresight. In workshops for parents of kids who happen to have physical disabilities, I stress four factors as vital in the development of their children. In order to focus on these qualities, it helps parents to project the child to age 25 in order to more effectively decide what abilities or skills he will need to meet his own needs. These four factors are Experience, Risk, Responsibility, and Socialization skills.

EXPERIENCE comes with living. We come to know about ourselves and others in a natural, unfolding process. Kids with disabilities often miss out on elemental experiences, such as riding a bike, helping weed the garden, or hiking into the wilderness. Some parents are often creative in enabling their child's participation. For instance, many have invested in specially designed bicycles or sleds. Some go on wilderness camping expeditions with companies that incorporate those with and without disabilities. More simply, feeling the rain, snow, or wind are all elemental experiences.

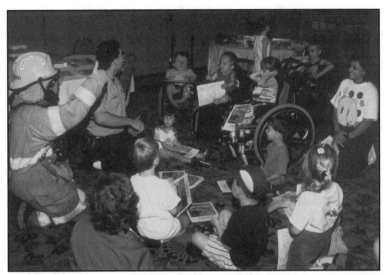

RISK TAKING is an important opportunity, often denied children with OI. It enables children to learn limits and the costs of consequences. This one factor is probably most frightening to the parents of kids with OI; that fear is to be duly appreciated! However, the element of risk is a path to building trust in one's self and one's abilities. (Note: At the 1996 National Osteogenesis Imperfecta Conference, a panel of young adults thanked their parents for allowing them to take risks and assess the results. These young adults felt this had enabled them to make better decisions as they grew older.) Some examples of risk taking are sending a child to sleep-away summer camp or saying "yes" to a request to go to a school dance.

RESPONSIBILITY goes with being a part of the human family. Yet there are many families where children with OI do not participate in contributing to the family. When children are needed in the family they feel valued and competent. This is accomplished through the assignment of tasks, such as digging dandelions, or being the official telephone answerer, or the dish wiper or the table setter at home. Responsibility to the larger community is learned through volunteering for a charitable or religious or political organization.

SOCIALIZATION is the give and take of normal interaction. It includes the shifting of the spotlight from one person to another. This shifting is not experienced by some children with OI; they are always in the spotlight and do not learn how to shift it to others. It also includes learning to deal on the same level with our peers. Sometimes children's experiences are primarily with adults and the medical community and they miss out on the important developmental peer interactions which can hinder adult psychosocial development. Another added element of socialization which kids with

OI need to learn is to build bridges via communication to others. This can be done through the use of a common bond such as an experience, an interest, or through humor, which is particularly effective. This bridge emphasizes similarities over differences.

Walking the Tightrope

The goal of all interventions is to maintain equilibrium within families so that they can function effectively in meeting all members' needs. The outcome of dealing with feelings and beginning to take control of life's variables (as much as that is possible) is families which have the balance, the expertise, and the supports to walk competently on the tightrope.

These families have flexibility to adapt and resiliency to deal with times of crisis and times of calm. They are able to restructure after a trauma, leaving themselves time for needed mourning. They are willing to reform the family structure when needed, redrawing family roles. They are also able to realign, changing positions of power and control, and to reassign tasks and responsibilities.

Families who walk the tightrope successfully have two other assets. One is a sense of hope which entails having a dream and some knowledge of how to attain the goal. The other asset is a sense of humor which allows the balancing of the tragedies and triumphs of life.

Some suggestions to help parents to keep the family system balanced include:

— Help them become expert on themselves and their families.
— Keep them informed.
— Help them to be open to new ways of dealing with problems.
— Encourage them to assume their roles as parents, recognizing their powers so as not to abuse them.
— Make sure that all members of the family are attended to.
— Encourage regular family meetings at which every member is heard and respectfully responded to.
— Assure them that "Perfect Families" are perfectly dull! Families are not meant to be perfect – they are moving, changing systems.
— Recognize but don't overemphasize disability.
— Suggest that every member of the family be a working member of the family. This builds competence, responsibility, and self esteem.
— Encourage families not to assign labels ("our saint", "the bad one") as they tend to stick.
— Recommend that parents take breathers. Suggest that couples take a night out or a weekend away to recharge their own marriages and bring new energy into the family.
— When really tough problems arise, families benefit from having

their own special family consultants – the wise older person, minister, priest, rabbi, counselor, psychologist, social worker, psychiatrist, etc.

— Help them identify their individual signals which tell them when they may fall off the tightrope. Precautions will help them to avoid the fall.

— Encourage the use of all available resources including books and periodicals, and information available on the Internet.

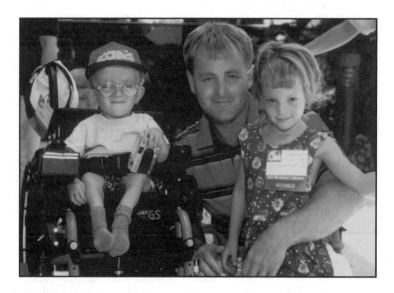

Conclusion

The process which proceeds from the birth of a child with OI can be the challenge to create triumph out of what some see as tragedy. In order to do that, families will require the psychic and physical energy, support, and resources to make wise and informed decisions. Physicians play an integral role in the lives of these families and have opportunities to help them validate feelings, confront fears, and to impart information and make referrals when appropriate.

Recommended Reading for Families and Professionals

Brazelton, Barry. On Becoming A Family: The Growth of Attachment. New York: Delacorte, 1981.

Brodin, J. "Children and Adolescents with Brittle Bones – Psycho-Social Aspects." Child: Care, Health, and Development. 1993, Vol. 19, 341-347.

Buscaglia, Leo. The Disabled and Their Parents. Thorofare, NJ: Charles B. Slack, Inc., 1975.

Cole, DEC. "Psychological Aspects of Osteogenesis Imperfecta: An Update." American Journal of Medical Genetics. 1993, Vol 42, 207-211.

Dobson, James. When God Doesn't Make Sense. Wheaton, Illinois: Tyndale House Publishers, Inc., 1993.

Featherstone, Helen. A Difference in the Family: Living With a Disabled Child. New York: Penguin Books, 1980.

Finston, Peggy, MD. Parenting Plus: Raising Children With Special Health Needs. New York: Dutton, 1990.

Kabat-Zinn, Jon. Full Catastrophe Living: Using the Wisdom of Your Body and Mind to Face Stress, Pain, and Illness. New York: Dell Publishing, 1990.

Kiersey, D.; Bates, M. Please Understand Me: Character and Temperament Types. Del Mar, CA: Gnosnology Books, 1984.

Kriegsman, K.H.; Rechsteiner, J.; Zaslow, E. Taking Charge: Teens Talk About Life and Physical Disability. Bethesda, MD: Woodbine House, Inc., 1992.

Kushner, Harold S. When All You've Ever Wanted Isn't Enough. New York: Pocketbooks, 1986.

Kushner, Harold S. When Bad Things Happen To Good People. New York: Schocken Books, 1981.

LeShan, Eda. "When Crises and Tragedies Occur." Grandparenting In A Changing World. New York: Newmarket Press, 1993.

Peck, M. Scott. The Road Less Traveled. New York: Simon and Schuster, 1978.

Powell, T.H.; Ogle, P.A. Brothers and Sisters: A Special Part of Exceptional Families. Baltimore, London: Paul H. Brooks Publishing, Co., 1985.

Siegel, Bernie S. Love, Medicine, and Miracles. New York: Harper and Row Publishers, 1986.

Simons, Robin. After the Tears: Parents Talk About Raising A Child With A Disability. San Diego, California: Harcourt, 1987.

Sullivan, Tom, Special Parent, Special Child. New York: G.P. Putnam's Sons, 1995.

Yancey, Phillip. Disappointment With God. New York: Harper Collins, Publishers, 1988.

Yancey, Phillip. Where is God When It Hurts? New York: Harper Collins, Publishers.

Chapter

21

Pain Management

by Douglas A. Friesen, MD

What is pain? Pain has been described as the perception of whatever causes discomfort at the time that it occurs. The International Association for the Study of Pain (I.A.S.P.) recently defined pain as "an unpleasant sensory and emotional experience associated with actual or potential tissue damage or described in terms of such."[1]

Pain is the most common presenting complaint which prompts a patient to see a physician. The past decade has brought an explosion in knowledge of the fundamental mechanisms of nociceptive transmission. Along with this knowledge has also been an unprecedented application of the theories to the development of innovative clinical treatment. Due to the pioneering efforts of anesthesiologist Dr. John Bonica, a modern field of pain management has been created. Progress continues with advances in research and clinical practice.

A brief overview will be given regarding the types of pain, then a brief discussion of acute pain and chronic pain. It is paramount to understand the concept of "total pain," describing how pain interferes with multiple dimensions of function. Pharmacological modalities along with physical and psychological methods, as well as the newest interventional treatment modalities for specific pain syndromes will be reviewed for common pain problems seen by physicians who treat patients with Osteogenesis Imperfecta (OI).

I. Classifications of Pain (by mechanism)

To begin the discussion of pain management, two types of pain need to be recognized: nociceptive and neuropathic pain. Nociceptive pain is separate and distinct from neuropathic pain, with nociceptive pain referring to a broad category of pain problems comprised of somatic and visceral pain.

Table 1
CLASSIFICATION OF PAIN

Nociceptive Pain	*Neuropathic Pain*
Somatic pain	Central pain
Visceral pain	Deafferentation pain

Nociceptive Pain

Nociceptive pain results from the sensations of simple and uncomplicated tissue injury (e.g. childbirth, trauma, fractures, surgery) and is usually associated with being painful. Nociceptive pain is subdivided into two classification: Somatic and Visceral. Transmission of pain impulses are on classical pain pathways with normal function of the peripheral nervous system. Nociceptive pain typically responds quickly to treatment with NSAIDS and opiates in a linear fashion.

Somatic pain Many types of stimuli such as mechanical, thermal, and chemical may initiate somatic pain by direct stimulation/activation of nociceptors in cutaneous and deep tissues. These symptoms are typically well localized and described as sharp/dull, aching, or gnawing (for example, bone metastasis or incisional pain). Somatic pain is sensitive to potent NSAIDS and opiates, and can be blocked, at least temporarily, by interruption of proximal pathways by local anesthetic blockade or surgery.

Visceral pain This pain results from the injury to sympathetically innervated internal organs. Mechanisms of injury differ from somatic since viscera are relatively insensitive to simple manipulation, cutting, and burning. However, abnormal distention or contraction of smooth muscle, rapid capsular stretch, ischemia, serosal and mucosal irritation by chemical stimuli, distention, traction or torsion of mesenteric attachments and vasculature, and necrosis will stimulate pain mechanisms. The typical visceral pain is characterized by being vague in distribution and quality, and described as deep, squeezing, aching, or pressure-like. At times it can also be associated with episodes of acute colicky or paroxys-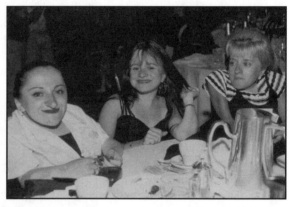mal episodes associated with nausea and vomiting; diaphoresis and alterations in blood pressure and pulse can also occur. Referred pain is usually present, with a phenomena of pain and hyperalgesia localized to deep or superficial areas distant to the source of pathology. Examples include: shoulder pain from hepatic origin, back pain from pancreatic or retroperitoneal pathology, upper extremity and neck pain from anginal origin, and knee pain from metastatic lesions of the hip. Visceral pain tends to be linearly responsive to opiates and can also be treated with potent NSAIDS and at times can be modified by proximal neural blockade.

Neuropathic Pain

This pain occurs in the presence of pathological functioning of the nervous system. Neuropathic pain can be subdivided into two groups, with the determination of central neuropathic vs. deafferentation pain relating to where the initial injury occurs. Depending upon whether the location of the causative lesion is located in the peripheral or central nervous system, this results in an aberrant somatosensory processing and "atypical pain." Neuropathic pain can be associated with objective neurological signs or altered sensation and is typically dysesthetic in nature. Dysesthetic neuropathic pain (an abnormal, unpleasant, either spontaneous or evoked sensation that produces pain) is described as burning, tingling, numbing, pressing, squeezing, and/or itching. Also associated with dysesthetic pain is a component of superimposed intermittent shock-like pain characterized by shooting, lancinating, or jolting in nature. Examples include: Herpes zoster, nerve impingement following surgery, brachial or lumbosacral plexopathy due to tumor invasion, radiation fibrosis, phantom limb phenomenon, diabetic neuropathy, and Reflex Sympathetic Dystrophy (RSD).

In general, neuropathic pain is more difficult to treat than nociceptive pain. It typically does not respond as favorably to opiates administered in the standard doses, even when given by neuroaxial routes of administration. At times these syndromes respond to centrally acting medications including heterocyclic anti-depressants, anticonvulsants, and oral local anesthetics (calcium channel blockers). A trial of three to four weeks is usually recommended to obtain an adequate dose-response relationship, however the response tends to be unpredictable. Ablative procedures or chemical neurolysis leading to further neurolysis can be beneficial.

II. Categories of Pain

In many acute/chronic painful disorders, the patients are correctly diagnosed and effectively treated, but there is an impressive body of evidence that suggests that all too many patients with severe post-operative and post-traumatic pain are not effectively treated. In addition to needless suffering, in many patients, unrelieved pain and perhaps the underlying pathophysiology cause it to progress to chronic pain. Since pain impairs one's ability to carry out a productive life, pain in general and particularly chronic pain is a serious economic problem as well as a major health problem.

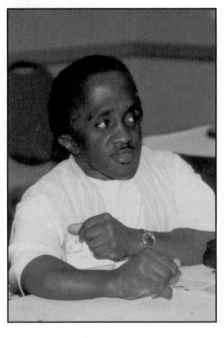

Acute Pain

Acute pain is usually characterized with a short duration and the pathology is discernible. There is normal functioning of both the peripheral and central nervous system, the prognosis is predictable, and the outcome is usually good.

At times, physicians have believed that adequate analgesic medication will either delay the diagnosis of a life threatening condition or have no clinical impact on treatment outcome. There is an impressive body of evidence which suggests that adequate pain relief will not delay the diagnosis of other pathological conditions. Also, adequate treatment of pain will also blunt adverse neuroendocrine responses as well as improve normal sleep and psychological profiles. If for no other reason but to prevent the emergence of a chronic pain syndrome, adequate analgesia should be a prominent consideration in the care of patients.

Chronic Pain

Many physicians use the term "chronic pain" to mean chronic benign pain while reserving the term "cancer pain" to encompass any cancer-related condition, either acute or chronic. It is obvious to the suffering patient that there is nothing benign about having a debilitating non-malignant pain. Chronic pain is the most frequent cause of suffering and disability in the world today. Chronic pain is defined as: a condition that persists one to three months beyond the time an expected acute pain or acute injury should subside. At times, the pathology is not known, and the prognosis is unpredictable. There can be other associated problems, and the treatment is multimodal.

III. Pain Syndromes and Osteogenesis Imperfecta

Osteogenesis Imperfecta is an inherited disorder characterized by bone fragility that is accompanied by other abnormalities of connective tissue. There can be associated conditions of acute and chronic pain associated with multiple fractures, vertebral collapse, severe metaphyseal osteoporosis, joint pain, osteoarthritis, contractures, deformity/malalignment, and recurrent abdominal pain.[2] The pain management of patients with OI, both adults and children requires adequate assessment and implementation of a regimen which should address the multifaceted presentation of acute and chronic pain. With the increased longevity of patients with OI, the incidences of pain syndromes relating to degenerative changes becomes more likely. An interdisciplinary approach to pain management should probably be instituted.

IV. Pain Management Modalities

Pharmacological

To provide adequate pain relief, the pharmacological principles of the medication need to be known. The prescriber should follow biopharmaceutical drug delivery models and know the pharmacodynamics. Recently (1986), the World Health Organizaion (WHO) convened a group of pain experts to develop an effective pain protocol. Two major guidelines were promoted as a result of this meeting: Strategies for Delivering Opioid regimens and the WHO Analgesic Ladder (Figure 1). A summary of the WHO "Strategies for Delivering Opioid Regimens for Acute Pain Relief"[3] (modified) includes:

• Individualize doses given at regular intervals to all patients, including infants and children (not "PRN").

• Know and understand the pharmacology of several analgesics and prescribe accordingly.

• Dosage according to physiological conditions and titrate medication accordingly. When changing medications, use equianalgesic doses.

• Placebo therapy should not be used in the assessment of pain conditions.

• Anticipate and recognize side effects early and treat appropriately.

• Address the patient's psychological state early in the therapy.

• Liberal use of analgesic adjuvants to help control pain.

Table 2

  Medications - use of adjuvants[10]
  • Nonsteroidal anti-inflammatory agents
  • Tricyclic antidepressants
  • Central acting medications (Carbamazepine)
  • Miscellaneous agents (fluoxetine, mexiletine)

The protocol of the WHO analgesic ladder uses common oral nonsteroidal analgesics and opiates to relieve mild, moderate, and severe cancer pain. As pain intensifies, patients are switched from nonopioid to opioid regimes (Figure 1). Titration of more potent opiates in addition to nonopioid analgesics and the use of adjuvant drugs improves the overall outcome. It was recently suggested that 90% of patients reported satisfactory or complete pain relief with this protocol.[4]

Opioid Analgesics

The use of opioid drugs for patients with nonmalignant pain continues to be controversial. The initial premise of traditional medicine that opioid use for nonmalignant pain was invariable, ineffective, and unsafe has been increasingly debated in the literature.[5,6,7] Even though the published literature continues to be limited, a growing number of studies cite clinical experience relating to long-term use and the discussion of concerns relating to addiction, tolerance, persistent side effects, and physical/psychosocial functioning. Many of these discussions are using the favorable clinical experience of long term opioid use in patients with a malignancy to reevaluate the current protocols for use in patients with nonmalignant pain.[8,9,10]

1.) **Opioid Activity.** Medications with morphine-like actions, natural and synthetic, have been referred to in a generic sense as opioid. Morphine continues to be the standard by which all other compounds with opioid activity that produce analgesia are measured. The most significant side effects of opioid medications include respiratory depression, analgesia,

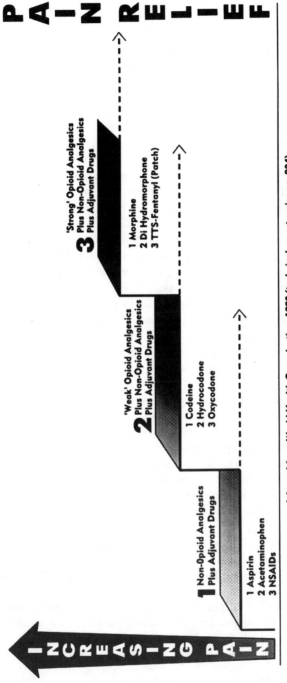

Adapted from World Health Organization, 1990 (technical report series no. 804)

This analgesic ladder presents a framework for treating patients effectively as the magnitude of pain increases. The pharmacological interventions are sequentially escalated to effectively manage the pain.

3 'Strong' Opioid Analgesics
Plus Non-Opioid Analgesics
Plus Adjuvant Drugs

1 Morphine
2 Di Hydromorphone
3 TTS-Fentanyl (Patch)

2 'Weak' Opioid Analgesics
Plus Non-Opioid Analgesics
Plus Adjuvant Drugs

1 Codeine
2 Hydrocodone
3 Oxycodone

1 Non-Opioid Analgesics
Plus Adjuvant Drugs

1 Aspirin
2 Acetaminophen
3 NSAIDs

PAIN RELIEF

INCREASING PAIN

Figure 1

drowsiness, mental clouding, dysphoria, pruritus, urinary retention, nausea, vomiting, changes in GI motility, and alterations of endocrine and autonomic nervous systems. Probably one of the most common and troubling side effects relates to the nauseant and emetic effects related to direct stimulation of the chemoreceptor trigger zone in the medulla.

2.) **Adverse Pharmacological Effects.** All opioid medications are metabolized by the liver. These medications should be used cautiously in patients with hepatic disease since cumulative effects and increased bioavailability may occur. Renal disease also can significantly effect the pharmocokinetic activity of those opiates which have an active metabolite (morphine, codeine, meperidine, and propoxyphene). Renal disease may cause the active metabolite to accumulate with the possibility of opioid overdose.

Great caution should be used in patients with compromised respiratory function: patients with emphysema, kyphoscoliosis, and obesity who demonstrate a reduction in respiratory reserve. The depressant effects on respiration can be disastrous to those patients who already demonstrate elevated levels of plasma CO_2 and then are less sensitive to the stimulation effects of an increase in plasma CO_2 caused by opioid use. Pulmonary edema has been reported in several patients receiving large doses.[11]

Allergic reactions to opioid medications is relatively uncommon. The usual manifestation is of skin rashes such as fixed eruptions, and urticaria can be observed. Anaphylactoid reactions are quite rare but have been reported after intravenous administration. Following an injection of some opioid medications, a skin wheal may be observed relating to the release of histamine.

Opioid medications are known to have interactions with various other medications. Phenothiazines, monoamine oxidase inhibitors, and tricyclic antidepressants can exaggerate and prolong the depressant effects of some opiates by a suspected supra-additive mechanism. Alterations in the rate of metabolic transformation or alterations in neurotransmitter may be the cause to this effect. There has also been reported to be an enhancement of the analgesic effect of opiates with the use of desipramine.

3.) **Critical Issues in the Treatment of Chronic Nonmalignant Pain with Opiate Therapy.** There are several critical issues in opioid therapy for patients with nonmalignant pain that need to be addressed.

a.) *Addiction.* Addiction and psychological dependence are synonymous and are characterized by the "compulsive use of a substance resulting in physical, psychological, and social harm to the user and continued use despite that harm."[12] Earlier studies have reported a substantial risk of addiction, but recent studies have correlated a much less risk of addiction.[13] However, proper guidelines need to be followed for the patient selection.[14] If addiction is suspected, a referral to a specialist in addiction medicine is recommended.

b.) *Physical dependence.* Physical dependence is distinct from addiction and involves the physiological state that is an inevitable result from the chronic use of opiates. This phenomenon is characterized by withdrawal (abstinence syndrome) following the abrupt discontinuation of the medicine, a substantial reduction of dose, and/or the use of a narcotic antagonist.

c.) *Tolerance.* Tolerance is described as an increase in the required doses over a period of time to achieve a given effect. This physiological state is an inevitable result of the chronic administration of opiates.

d.) *Pseudoaddiction.* An iatrogenic syndrome that is characterized by addictive-like behavior is called pseudoaddiction. This may be actually a legitimate response to the inadequate treatment of pain.

Nerve Blocks

There are a myriad of conditions that can be treated with various nerve blocks. The most common presenting symptom is "low back pain" (LBP). Following a thorough history, physical examination, and the appropriate imaging studies and possibly nerve conduction studies, various nerve blocks can be performed. These can include epidural steroid injections, trigger point injections, sciatic nerve blocks, piriformis nerve blocks, lumbar plexus blocks, facet joint injections (or blocking the lumber medial branch injections), and lumbar sympathetic blocks.

Epidural steroid injections Following conservative management with minimal change in symptoms, the next step in therapy is an epidural steroid injection (ESI). Clearly, not every patient with LBP is a candidate nor will demonstrate benefit form this technique. This procedure should be usually limited to those who demonstrate radicular symptoms. A reasonable success rate of 60 to 70% can be expected from radicular pain and acute herniated discs in the lumbar, thoracic, and cervical levels.[15,16,17,18,19]

Patients with OI who are candidates for ESI include:
• those with an acute herniated disc after four to six weeks of other therapy,
• patients with acute pain and having chronic LBP syndrome with a flare-up of symptoms that have radiculoid features and a poor response to other conservative measures after four to six weeks,
• those with a history of chronic radicular pain and a corresponding sensory change who fail at conservative therapy, and
• motivated patients with postural LBP with radiculoid features (i.e. the patient with a bulging disc).

Other candidates for ESI:
• patients with metastatic carcinoma in whom tumor infiltration of the nerve roots cause a radicular pain,
• some selected patients with LBP, with ESI as part of a comprehensive pain management program, and
• selected patients with spinal stenosis.[20]

Patients with OI who have scoliosis present a challenge for placement of ESI. One must not only consider the spinal curvature, but also the rotational changes in the lumbar vertebral column. The literature acknowledges that ESI has relatively few side-effects and complications, and that the most common complications were related not to the steroid but the technical aspects of the procedure.[21]

Trigger point injections Dramatic results can be obtained with using trigger point injections into the affected areas of persons with fibromyalgia and myofascial pain syndrome. Saline, local anesthetic, corticosteroid, and NSAIDS have all been successfully used as injectates.

Interventional Modalities

Transcutaneous nerve stimulation (TENS) has been available for many years, and now there are two new interventional techniques modalities for treatment of intractable pain: Spinal Cord Stimulation and an Implantable Infusion System. These systems can be effective for patients who are unresponsive to conservative measures, who experience minimal relief and/or unmanageable side effects with increasing doses of narcotics or whose pain condition is not surgically correctable.

Transcutaneous nerve stimulation (TENS) TENS utilizes peripheral stimulation of afferent fibers to control pain. Selective stimulation of primary afferent nerve fibers has been reported to control pain refractory to conventional methods in 30% of patients with chronic pain and 60% of patients with acute pain.[23]

Spinal cord stimulation (SCS) The initial technology was developed in the 1960's with pacemaker research, with the first implantable SCS lead placement performed in 1974. This system involves a power source, a conductor, and then a stimulating electrode. The target is the epidural space of the spinal cord in the distribution of the pain. SCS primarily involves treatment of neuropathic pain and pain mediated by NMDA receptors.

This type of pain is usually resistant to usual clinical doses of opioids. The SCS in nondestructive, nonaddictive, and reversible; the patient undergoes a trial period before implantation occurs. Careful selection is essential in determining a successful outcome. Patients who respond

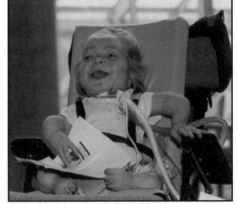

well include those with: Postherpetic neuralgia, peripheral neuropathies/ causalgias, mononeuropathies, plexopathies, RSD, "failed back syndrome," adhesive arachnoiditis, ischemic pain of vascular origin, and phantom limb syndrome. These patients have failed conventional therapy and are not candidates for further surgical correction and demonstrate predominantly radicular extremity pain.

When SCS is appropriately used, the success rate is 60 to 70% with a good to excellent rating on pain relief. This allows a substantial reduction in analgesic intake, and improved activity. Most importantly, patients report they are able to resume a normal life-style, enjoy psychological benefits, and have an overall improvement in the quality of life. Several prospective, randomized studies have indicated the success the spinal cord stimulation for failed back surgery syndrome.[24,25]

Implantable Infusion Systems This treatment modality is available for patients who have not received adequate pain relief from more conventional therapies and primarily have nociceptive pain. Examples include patients with OI who also have bone pain, pain elicited by tissue injury, cancer pain, axial somatic pain, and chronic pancreatitis. However, this treatment modality should only be considered when all other treatment modalities have failed.

After a trial screening to determine the effectiveness of intrathecal narcotics, the pump is surgically implanted in the abdominal wall, with a catheter placement in the subarachnoid space in the lumbar regions and directed cephalad to the lower thoracic levels. The Synchromed drug infusion pump by Medtronic is a micro infusion system which provides continuous intrathecal dosage, thus eliminating the "peaks and valleys" associated with oral or intramuscular medication. The infusion system can be programmed with various infusion doses at different times during a 24 hour period. The infusion dose can be easily adjusted through the use of a specialized portable laptop computer programmer which transmits instruction to the implanted pump by radiotelemetry. The clinician uses the programmer to set and adjust the dosage, drug flow rate, and other variables relating to dosing patterns throughout the day. The pump has a reservoir holding 18 cubic centimeters which can be refilled percutaneously with a needle and a syringe.

The intrathecal delivery of morphine in clinical studies has provided good pain relief in 80 to 87% of carefully screened patients who have failed conventional therapy. These studies suggest that a significant reduction in severe intractable pain can be obtained with few complications and low incidence of tolerance. Many patients have also experienced a significant reduction in systemic narcotics.[26,27,28] These studies demonstrate a significant reduction in severe intractable pain with few complications and low incidence of tolerance.

The use of intrathecal drug delivery for patients for both malignant and nonmalignant pain has proven to be successful. In the treatment of cancer pain, the goal of pain relief clearly justifies the costly invasive intrathecal opioid infusion system. However, the treatment of chronic nonmalignant benign pain involves special considerations. These considerations are by no means trivial and should be taken into careful consideration before embarking on this treatment modality. The goal in nonmalignant pain extends beyond pain control, but also encompasses an increased capacity to work as well as an improvement in psychological and social performance.

Physical Modalities

Many patients with pain due to disease, injury, or loss of body function can obtain a reduction in acute pain and relieve subacute/chronic pain over an extended time period with physical modalities. The three primary goals of physical therapy in the control of pain have been described by Yeh.[29] These include:

1.) to make an assessment of the most effective modalities to decrease and control the patient's pain,

2.) after determination of any dysfunction in an initial assessment, to use modalities to correct the dysfunction, and

3.) to restore the patient's confidence in their ability to function without the risk of reinjury or exacerbation of their pain. The physical modalities team approach should include the physiatrist, neurologist, orthopaedist, physical therapist, vocational therapist, and occupational therapist.

Psychological Interventions

Patients who suffer from chronic pain may need and could benefit from a psychological evaluation. There is a wide variability to the pain threshold and just as great a diversity of idiosyncratic responses to this pain. The global response is dictated by our individual personality traits and inclinations, can be tempered or aggravated by any emotional or psychological problems, and can also be influenced by economic, social, behavioral, and financial considerations. In general, even in patients with a strong constitution, unresolved chronic pain will lead to varying degrees of frustration, anger, irritability, and depression.

There currently are many psychological investigative tools: MMPI, Multi-axial Assessment of Pain (MAP), Beck Depression Test, McGil pain questionnaire, etc. These can provide an initial assessment and lead to further psychological interventions such as individual counseling, biofeedback, operant conditioning, group therapy, behavioral therapy, and relaxation therapy.

Multi-Disciplinary Approach

In an attempt to provide the maximum benefit for patients who have OI with long-term chronic pain, it is paramount that this pain is best managed under the auspices of a multi-disciplinary, multi-modal approach. Not only should the acute/chronic pain aspects of their disease be addressed pharmacologically, but careful consideration should be made to the emotional, social, and psychological aspects of patients with OI.

V. Conclusion

Albert Schweitzer, a great humanitarian, physician, and Nobel Laureate, wrote a description of the obligation and privilege of the physician to relieve pain. In 1931, after spending 20 years working in an African jungle, he wrote this regarding the nature of pain in his book On the Edge of the Primeval Forest: "We must all die. But that I can save him from days of torture, that is what I feel as my great and ever new privilege. Pain is a more terrible lord of mankind than even death itself."

Chronic pain is one of the most important health problems in industrialized nations. The economic cost to society is immeasurable. Patients should have treatment with the concept of "Total Pain" – how pain interferes with multiple dimensions of function. We must all recognize that pain is not an unidimensional phenomenon, assessment and treatment should focus on the pain problems' multiple determinants, and the treatment at times will be multi-modal. This will occasionally require a multi-disciplinary approach with the use of specialists in medical, psychological, and rehabilitative fields for adequate treatment. The goal for treatment of these patients is effective therapy that will not only reduce or remove the pain, but will also achieve mental well-being and an improvement in physiological function.

References
[1] Mersky H, Bogduk N. (eds). Classification of Chronic Pain, ed. 2, IASP Press. Seattle, 1994.
[2] Lee JH. Gastrointestinal problems in patients who have type III osteogenesis imperfecta. J of Bone and Joint Surgery. September 1995;77A:1252-1356.
[3] World Health Organization, Technical report series no. 804, 1990.
[4] Lema MJ. Cancer pain management: An overview of current therapeutic regimens. Seminars in Anesthesia. 1993;12:109-117.
[5] Brena SF. Opiates in nonmalignant pain: Questions in search of answers. Clin J Pain, 1991;7:342-345.
[6] Chabal C, et. al. Narcotics for chronic pain: Yes or no? A useless dichotomy. APS Journal, 1992;1:276-281.
[7] Portenoy RK. Opioid therapy for nonmalignant pain. J Pain Symptom Manage, 1990;5:S46-S62.
[8] Jorgensen L, et. al. Treatment of cancer pain patients in a multi disciplinary pain clinic. The Pain Clinic, 1990;3:83-89.
[9] Schug SA. Cancer pain management according to WHO analgesic guidelines. J Symptom Manage, 1990;5:27-32.
[10] Ventafridda V. A validation study of the WHO method for cancer pain relief. Cancer, 1987;59: 850-856.
[11] Bruera, Miller. Non-cardiogenic pulmonary edema after narcotic treatment for cancer pain. Pain, 1989;39:297-300.
[12] Rinaldi RC. Classification and standardization of substance abuse terminology. JAMA, 1988;259:555-557.
[13] Porter J. Addiction rare in patients treated with narcotics. N Engl J Med, 1980;302:123.
[14] Porteroy RK. Opioid therapy for chronic nonmalignant pain: A review of the clinical issues. J Pain Symptom Manage, 1996;11:203-217.

[15] Berman AT, et. al. The effects of epidural injections of local anesthetic and corticosteroid on patients with lumbosciatic pain. Clin Ortho Rel Res, 1984;188:144-51.

[16] Wheeler AH. Diagnosis and treatment of LBP and sciatica. American Family Physician, 1995;52(5): 1333-41.

[17] Ellenburg MR. Cervical radiculopathy. Arch Phy Med Rehabil, 1994;75(3):342-52.

[18] Bush K. LBP and sciatica. Br J Hosp Med, 1994;51(5):216-21.

[19] Ferrante FM, Wilson SP, et. al. Clinical classification as a predicator of therapeutic outcome after cervical epidural steroid injection. Spine, 1993;18(6):730-36.

[20] Hacobian A. Treatment of SS with ESI, an outcome study. (Harvard University) Annual meeting of the American Society of Regional Anesthesia, March, 1995.

[21] Abrams S, O'Connor T. Complications associated with epidural steroid injections. Regional Anesthesia, 1996;21(2):149-162.

[22] Clauw D. Fibromyalgia. More than just a musculoskeletal disease. Amer Fam Phys, 1995;52(3):843-851.

[23] Wall, Melzick. Stimulation-induced analgesia: TENS and vibration. Textbook of Pain, 1994;1191-1208.

[24] North RB, Kidd DH, Lee MS, Piantodosi S. A prospective, randomized study of spinal cord stimulation versus reoperation for failed back surgery syndrome: Initial results. Stereotact Funct Neurosurgery, 1994;62:267-72.

[25] Burchiel KJ. Prognostic factors of spinal cord stimulator for chronic back and leg pain. Neurosurgery, 1995;36:1101-1111.

[26] Kanoff R. Intraspinal delivery of implantable infusion systems. JAOA, 1994;487-93.

[27] Hassenbusch S. Constant infusion of morphine for intractable cancer pain using an implanted pump. J of Neurosurgery, 1990;73:405-409.

[28] Penn R. Chronic intrathecal morphine for intractable pain. J of Neurosurgery, 1987;192-86.

[29] Yeh C, et. al. Physical therapy: Evaluation and treatment of chronic pain. Evaluation and Treatment of Chronic Pain, 1985;251-261.

[30] Practice Guidelines for Cancer Pain Management – A report by the American Society of Anesthesiologists Task Force on Pain Management, Cancer Pain Section. Anesthesiology, 1996;84:1243-57.

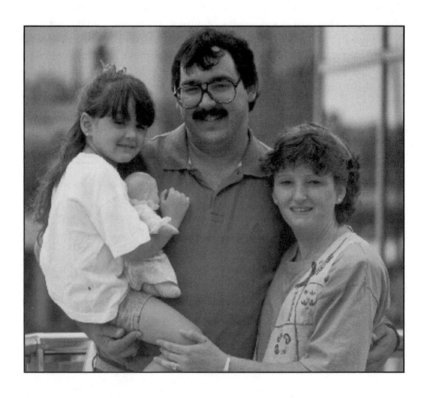

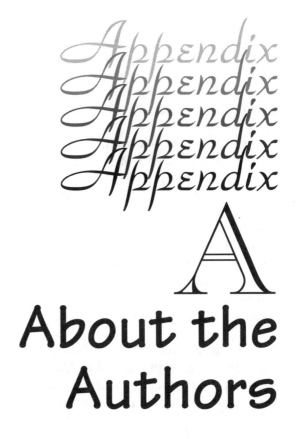

About the
Authors

Patrick Agnew, DPM, is a Fellow of the American College of Foot and Ankle Surgeons and a Fellow of the American College of Foot and Ankle Pediatrics. He has a private podiatric practice in Virginia Beach, Virginia, as well as being an associate professor at Eastern Virginia Graduate School of Medicine and Podopediatrics

Director of the Norfolk Community Hospital Podiatric Residency. He has a special interest in persons, especially children, with connective tissue disorders, serving on the Medical Advisory Panel of the Ehlers-Danlos National Foundation.

G. Hossein Almassi, MD, is Associate Professor of Cardiothoracic Surgery at the Medical College of Wisconsin and Chief of Cardiothoracic Surgery Section, Zablocki V.A. Medical Center, Milwaukee, Wisconsin. A 1976 graduate from Shiraz University School of Medicine in Iran, his general surgical training was performed at the University of Chicago and the University of Illinois, Metropolitan Group Hospitals Program in Chicago. He subsequently obtained training in Cardiothoracic Surgery at the Medical College of Wisconsin where he is currently practicing adult cardiac and aortic surgery. He has published a manuscript on the cardiac surgery of a patient with OI.

Anna August, MD, is a Pediatrician and Neonatologist at Washington University School of Medicine in St. Louis, Missouri. She completed her undergraduate training and medical studies at the University of Alabama followed by a pediatric residency at the University of Cincinnati and Children's Hospital Medical Center. Following residency, Dr. August completed a fellowship program in Neonatology at St. Louis Children's Hospital at Washington University School of Medicine. She is currently a member of the faculty at Washington University where she has an appointment as Assistant Professor of Pediatrics. In addition to caring for newborns in the Intensive Care Unit, she is Director of the Newborn Medicine Follow-up Clinic, which provides comprehensive care to high risk neonates after discharge from the hospital. Dr. August has been involved in the care of infants with OI both in the delivery room and the NICU.

M. Ines Boechat, MD, is a Professor of Radiology and Pediatrics at the UCLA School of Medicine. She is the Chief of Pediatric Radiology at UCLA Children's Hospital and the Director of the Pediatric Radiology Fellowship Program at the same institution. She did her training in Pediatric Radiology at Children's Hospital Medical Center in Boston and at UCLA, where she has been practicing since 1982. Dr. Boechat evaluates the radiographs of children with

OI seen in the pediatric orthopaedic clinic and also works with the geneticist in the initial work up of affected children.

Peter H. Byers, MD, is an Internist and Medical Geneticist. He received his undergraduate education at Reed College, Portland, Oregon, and his medical degree from Case Western University, Cleveland, Ohio. He has been at the University of Washington in Seattle since 1974 where he is Professor and Director of the Medical Genetics Clinic. He served as chairman of the Medical Advisory Council of the Osteogenesis Imperfecta Foundation from 1990 until 1995. Dr. Byers has authored multiple manuscripts about OI for journals and textbooks, and he is well known for the research his laboratory performs on the skin cells of persons with OI.

Jay W. Carlson, DO, MS, is the Chief of the Department of Obstetrics and Gynecology at William Beaumont Army Medical Center, El Paso, Texas, that serves as the military referral center for high risk obstetrics for West Texas, New Mexico, and Arizona. As such, he has had the opportunity to care for patients with OI and has previously published on the subject of pregnancy and OI.

Holly Lea Cintas, PhD, is Physical Therapy Research Coordinator in the Rehabilitation Medicine Department at the Clinical Center, National Institutes of Health, Bethesda, Maryland. She is a board certified pediatric physical therapist and a developmental psychologist who co-authored The Handbook of Pediatric Physical Therapy in 1995. Formerly Director of Physical Therapy at Children's Hospital of Philadelphia, her experience with OI has been primarily at the NIH in collaboration with Dr. Lynn Gerber.

Garrett H. C. Colmorgen, MD, is Senior Attending Physician and Chairman of the Special Deliveries Clinical Advisory Board at the Medical Center of Delaware in Wilmington, Delaware. He received a BS in chemistry, biochemistry, and molecular biology from Centre College of Kentucky and his MD from the College of Medicine and Dentistry of New Jersey, New Jersey Medical School. He completed a residency in obstetrics and gynecology at Monmouth Medical Center in Long Branch, New Jersey, and a fellowship in Maternal-Fetal Medicine at Pennsylvania Hospital in Philadelphia, Pennsylvania.

Robert J. Feigal, DDS, PhD, presently is Professor and Director of Pediatric Dentistry, Department of Orthodontics and Pediatric Dentistry, University of Michigan. His dental, specialty, and PhD training was completed at the University of Minnesota where he subsequently served as graduate program director and chairman of Pediatric Dentistry. Dr. Feigal has treated patients with OI at both university settings and in private practice with Dr. Kurt King.

Douglas A. Friesen, MD, is an Anesthesiologist who is the medical director of Midwest Pain Management Center, P.A., in Hutchinson, Kansas. The pain clinic provides pain management services for central and western Kansas. He is a diplomate of the American Academy of Pain Management. He has undergraduate degrees in Biology and Pharmacy and a medical degree from the University of Kansas. After a surgical internship, he completed his residency in anesthesiology from the University of Kansas Medical School, Wichita. He has been in private practice in Hutchinson for ten years.

Lynn H. Gerber, MD, is Chief, Rehabilitation Medicine Department, Clinical Center, National Institutes of Health. She is board certified in Internal Medicine, Rheumatology, and Physical Medicine and Rehabilitation. She has participated in programs sponsored by the National Institute of Child Health and Human Development at NIH studying the biochemical and genetic aspects of OI. Her interests include understanding the efficacy of bracing for children with OI.

Thomas N. Hangartner, PhD, is a native of Switzerland. He received his doctorate in experimental physics at the Swiss Federal Institute of Technology in Zurich. From 1979 to 1985, he performed research at The University of Alberta in Edmonton, Canada. Since 1986, he has been at Wright State University and Miami Valley Hospital in Dayton, Ohio. His research interests center around the non-invasive, quantitative evaluation of bone. He has developed special computed tomography methods to precisely measure bone density, and the currently used scanner, the OsteoQuant®, is unique in the United States. For several years now, he has evaluated patients with unexplained multiple fractures not only from the Dayton area, but from all over the country.

Donna King, PhD, studied Developmental Biology at the University of Cincinnati. She is currently on the faculty at The Chicago Medical School, where she teaches and conducts research on the effects of growth hormone on bones of mice (including mouse models of OI). She is hopeful that gene therapy strategies will be developed eventually to strengthen and maintain the bones of young patients with OI. She emphasizes the importance of basic research using animals to achieve that goal.

Kurt J. King, DDS, MS, graduated from the University of Michigan with a DDS and a MSD in pediatric dentistry. For ten years, he was the director of the Department of Dentistry at the Minneapolis Children's Hospital Residency Program. Currently in private pediatric dentistry practice, he has provided dental care for several children with OI as well as authoring several articles regarding the care of children with disabilities.

Kay Harris Kriegsman, PhD, is a Psychologist in private practice in Bethesda, Maryland. She works with individuals with and without physical disabilities. Co-director of the HOW Conference (a yearly conference for teenagers with physical disabilities, their parents, and their teenaged siblings), Dr. Kriegsman conducts workshops nationally for parents of children with disabilities, women with disabilities, and teenagers and young adults with disabilities. Co-author of <u>Taking Charge: Teens Talk About Life and Physical Disability</u>, Dr. Kriegsman has also made professional presentations and written professional journal articles on women, college students, and teens with physical disabilities. She is married and has two married children and one grandson.

Roger W. Lidman, MD, earned his AB at Duke University and MD at the Johns Hopkins University. He served his internship and residency at Vanderbilt University. He received his rheumatology training at Vanderbilt and at the Medical University of South Carolina, then returned to the clinical faculty at Vanderbilt. Since 1981, he has practiced with The Center for Arthritis and Rheumatic Disease in Virginia Beach, Virginia, and is Clinical Associate Professor of Medicine at the Eastern Virginia Medical School. His clinical contacts with patients who have OI date to his fellowship training.

G. Larry Maxwell, MD, received his undergraduate degree with honors from the University of North Carolina at Wilmington. He earned his MD with honors from the University of North Carolina School of Medicine. After joining the Army, he trained in an obstetrics and gynecology internship and residency at William Beaumont Army Medical Center in El Paso, Texas. During his training, he received numerous awards for his research. For the past two years, Dr. Maxwell has practiced as a General Obstetrician and Gynecologist in Fort Knox, Kentucky. He will be starting a fellowship in Gynecological Oncology at Duke University in July, 1997.

C. Michael Reing, MD, is a board certified Orthopaedic Surgeon and a board certified Pediatrician. He is clinical assistant professor for orthopaedic surgery at Georgetown University and clinical assistant professor for pediatrics at the University of Virginia. Since his fellowship at Vanderbilt University in pediatric orthopaedics, he has been practicing pediatric orthopaedics and spinal surgery at Fairfax Hospital in Virginia where he is chief of pediatric orthopaedics and spine surgery at the Fairfax Hospital for Children. He is the clinical consultant for Osteogenesis Imperfecta at the National Institutes of Health and is currently involved in research protocols at the National Institutes of Health for Osteogenesis Imperfecta and intramedullary rodding in Osteogenesis Imperfecta.

Jay Shapiro, MD, is a graduate of Franklin and Marshall College and the Boston University School of Medicine. He is Professor of Medicine at Johns Hopkins University where he directs the Osteoporosis Clinic on the Johns Hopkins Bayview Research Campus. For several years, Dr. Shapiro has conducted both basic and clinical research on the subject of Osteogenesis Imperfecta. Dr. Shapiro and his colleagues have extensively studied the metabolism of bone cells from patients with OI and related metabolic bone disorders. This research has pointed to the significant effects type I collagen mutations have on the metabolism of bone cells and the development of structurally sound bone.

Chester H. Sharps, MD, graduated with a BS in Biology from David Lipscomb College in Nashville, Tennessee. He received his medical training at Hahnemann Medical School in Philadelphia, Pennsylvania, then went on to complete a residency in Orthopaedic

Surgery at Hahnemann University in Philadelphia. For fellowship training in pediatric orthopaedics, he went to the Alfred I. DuPont Institute in Wilmington, Delaware. Dr. Sharps has been practicing pediatric orthopaedics in Richmond, Virginia, since 1985 and has treated many patients with OI.

Paul D. Sponseller, MD, grew up in Ann Arbor, Michigan, and attended undergraduate and medical school at the University of Michigan. He completed orthopaedic residency at the University of Wisconsin, Madison. His fellowship in Pediatric Orthopaedics and Pediatric Spine Surgery was at the Children's Hospital and Harvard Medical School, Boston. Dr. Sponseller has been on the faculty at Johns Hopkins for ten years. His interest in OI has been fostered by the strong genetics department at Johns Hopkins and by his contact with Dr. Jay Shapiro.

Robert Steiner, MD, is a Pediatrician and Medical Geneticist at Oregon Health Sciences University (OHSU) in Portland, Oregon. He completed his undergraduate and medical studies at the University of Wisconsin. He went on to complete a residency in Pediatrics at the University of Cincinnati and Children's Hospital Medical Center. After residency, Dr. Steiner pursued fellowship training in Medical Genetics at the University of Washington in Seattle where he worked in the laboratory of Dr. Peter Byers. His research focused on the molecular genetic basis of OI and the differentiation of OI from child abuse. Upon completion of fellowship, Dr. Steiner accepted a position as Instructor of Pediatrics at Washington University School of Medicine where, among other duties, he worked with Dr. Michael Whyte at Shiners Hospital in St. Louis seeing children with OI. After three years in St. Louis, Dr. Steiner left for a position as Assistant Professor of Pediatrics and Molecular & Medical Genetics. Currently he sees children with OI at Shriners Hospital for Crippled Children in Portland and at OHSU Hospital and the Child Development and Rehabilitation Center at OHSU. He currently is involved in research evaluating a possible treatment for OI.

David M. Vernick, MD, is Assistant Professor of Otology and Laryngology at Harvard Medical School. He graduated from Johns Hopkins Medical School, then was a surgical intern and assistant resident in surgery at George Washington Hospital in Washington,

D.C. He was a resident in otolaryngology at Massachusetts Eye and Ear Infirmary in Boston, and he has also completed fellowships in otology and otolaryngology. A prolific writer and lecturer, he has served on the Osteogenesis Imperfecta Foundation Medical Advisory Committee since 1993.

Priscilla Ridgway Wacaster, MD, graduated with a BA in mathematics from Anderson University, Anderson, Indiana, and then went to medical school at the University of Arkansas for Medical Sciences, Little Rock, Arkansas. She completed an internship in family medicine at Riverside Regional Medical Center, Newport News, Virginia, then left the program to care for her son. Dr. Wacaster continues to live in Newport News, Virginia, and works part-time for Sentara Health Care Centers, providing urgent care. She is a strong advocate of early intervention, serving on the Local Intraagency Coordinating Council for early intervention in her area. She is the leader of the Virginia OI Support Group. Both Dr. Wacaster and her son have OI Type I.

Nancy B. White, OT, an orthopaedic technologist, is currently preparing to sit for certification with the National Board of Certification of Orthopaedic Technologists. She is in an independent study program with the guidance of Tom Byrne, MD, with Grossmont College in El Cajon, California. She is receiving her clinical training under Daniel F. Kinar, MD, an orthopaedic surgeon in Kingsport, Tennessee. She is a member of the National Association of Orthopaedic Technologists and serves on the speakers bureau of the Osteogenesis Imperfecta Foundation. She also serves as the vice-chairman of the Mayors Advisory Council for the Handicapped in Kingsport, Tennessee and is on the board of directors for Parents and Advocates for Children in Education (P.A.C.E.) Partnership. She has an 11 year old son with Osteogenesis Imperfecta, Type IV.

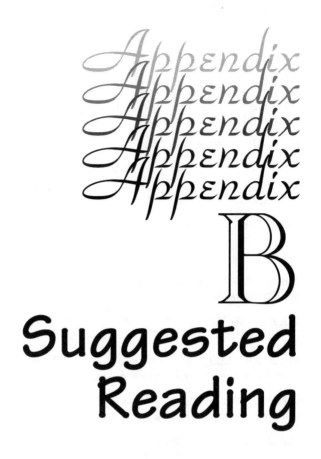

Appendix B

Suggested Reading

For Children

<u>**Arnie and the New Kid**</u> by N. Carlson. Published by The Trumpet Club, N.Y. Grades K to 3.

A Very Special Critter by G. and M. Mayer. Published by Western Pub. Co., Racine, Wisconsin. Preschool to grade 3.

How It Feels To Live With A Physical Disability by Jill Krementz. Published by Simon & Shuster, N.Y. Teenagers.

Howie Helps Himself by Joan Fassler. Published by Albert Whitman & Co., Chicago, Illinois. Preschool.

Like It Is: Facts and Feelings About Handicaps From Kids Who Know by James Stanfield. Published by Walker & Co., N.Y. Teenagers.

Living With A Brother or Sister With Special Needs: A Book for Sibs by D.J. Meyer, P.V. Vadasy, and R.R. Fewell. Published by University of Washington Press, Seattle, Washington. Ages 9 and up.

Mark's Wheelchair Adventure by Camilia Jessell. Published by Methuen, N.Y. Preschool to grade 3.

My Brother Matthew by M. Thompson. Published by Woodbine House, Bethesda, Maryland. Grades 1 to 5. Great for siblings.

My Friend Leslie by M. B. Rosenberg. Published by Lothrop, Lee, & Shepard, N.Y. Preschool to grade 3.

On Our Own Terms by Thomas Bergman. Published by Gareth Stevens Children's Books, Milwaukee, Wisconsin. Grades K to 3.

Our Teacher in a Wheelchair by Mary Ellen Powers. Published by Albert Whitman & Co., Chicago, Illinois. Ages 4 to 7.

Overcoming Disability by B.R. Ward. Published by Franklin Watts, N.Y. Grades 1 to 5.

Princess Pooh by Kathleen Muldoon. Published by Albert Whitman & Co., Grove, Illinois. Grades K to 3.

Someone Special Just Like You by T. Brown. Published by Henry Holt & Co., N.Y. Ages 3 to 7.

Taking Charge: Teens Talk About Life and Physical Disability by K.H. Kriegsman, J. D'Amura-Rechsteiner, and E.L. Zaslow. Published by Woodbine House, Inc., Bethesda, Maryland. Teenagers.

The Little Lame Prince by Rosemary Wells. Published by Dial Books for Young Readers, N.Y. Ages 5 to 12.

Treasures of the Snow by Patricia St. John. Published by Moody Press, Chicago, Illinois. Grades 4 to 7.

What If You Couldn't:... by Janet Kamien. Published by Charles Scribner's Sons, Old Tappan, New Jersey. Grades K to 3.

Wheelchair Champions by Harriet May Savitz. Published by Harper and Row, N.Y. Grades 1 to 6.

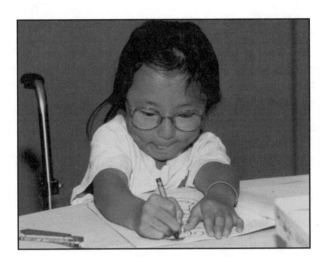

For Adults

A Difference in the Family: Living With a Disabled Child by Helen Featherstone. Published by Penguin Books, N.Y.

After the Tears: Parents Talk About Raising A Child With A Disability by Robin Simons. Published by Harcourt, San Diego, California. *An excellent book for new parents.*

Brothers and Sisters: A Special Part of Exceptional Families by T.H. Powell, and P.A. Ogle. Published by Paul H. Brooks Publishing, Co., Baltimore, Maryland.

Disappointment With God by Phillip Yancey. Published by Harper Collins, Publishers, N.Y.

From the Heart: On Being the Mother of a Child With Special Needs edited by Jayne D. B. Marsh. Published by Woodbine House, Bethesda, Maryland. *This book will make you laugh and make you cry, and it should be read by every mother of children with disabilities. It covers all age children, newborn to teenager.*

Full Catastrophe Living: Using the Wisdom of Your Body and Mind to Face Stress, Pain, and Illness by Jon Kabat-Zinn. Published by Dell Publishing, N.Y.

Love, Medicine, and Miracles by Bernie S. Siegel. Published by Harper and Row Publishers, N.Y.

No Pity by Joseph Shapiro. Published by Random House, N.Y. *A history of the Disability Rights Movement and how it is changing America.*

On Becoming A Family: The Growth of Attachment by Barry Brazelton, MD. Published by Delacorte, N.Y. *This has an especially good chapter about a family with a premature child in a NICU.*

Parenting Plus: Raising Children With Special Health Needs by Peggy Finston, MD. Published by Dutton, N.Y. *An excellent book by a psychiatrist who has two children with special health needs.*

Please Understand Me: Character and Temperament Types by D. Kiersey and M. Bates. Published by Gnosnology Books, Del Mar, California.

Special Parent, Special Child by Tom Sullivan. Published by G.P. Putnam's Sons, N.Y. *Parents share their trials and triumphs. An excellent book for parents with children in kindergarten through third grades.*

The Disabled and Their Parents by Leo Buscaglia. Published by Charles B. Slack, Inc., Thorofare, New Jersey.

The Road Less Traveled by M. Scott Peck. Published by Simon and Schuster, N.Y.

Uncommon Fathers: Reflections on Raising a Child With A Disability edited by Donald Meyer. Published by Woodbine House, Bethesda, Maryland. *Essays by fathers of children with disabilities.*

When All You've Ever Wanted Isn't Enough by Harold S. Kushner. Published by Pocketbooks, N.Y.

When Bad Things Happen To Good People by Harold S. Kushner. Published by Schocken Books, N.Y.

When God Doesn't Make Sense by James Dobson. Published by Tyndale House Publishers, Inc., Wheaton, Illinois. *Help for holding onto faith in God when your world is falling apart.*

Where is God When It Hurts? by Phillip Yancey. Published by Harper Collins, Publishers, N.Y.

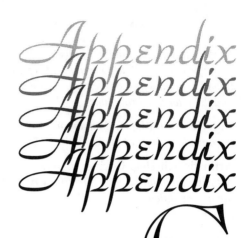

Appendix C

Glossary of Selected Terms

Allele: *the copy of a gene which one receives from one parent. A person's genetic code contains two alleles, or copies, of each gene, one from each parent.*

Amino Acids: *molecules which form the building blocks of a protein. DNA code determines the number and sequence of amino acids.*

Amphiarthrodial Joints: *joints lined with thicker fibrocartilage generally in the form of disc-like material that separates bone ends that are themselves joined by ligamentous structures. An example would be the symphysis pubis and the intervertebral joints.*

Anserine Bursitis: *inflammation of a small bursa (fluid filled sac) at the inframedial aspect of the knee.*

Arthritis Self-Help Course: *a program sponsored by local chapters of the Arthritis Foundation which instructs patients and their families in exercise, dietary modifications, and other strategies to improve the quality of life for patients with arthritis.*

Bivalve Cast: *cast that is split in half (clam-shelled) by cuts made on opposite sides of the cast to release pressure or allow removal and reapplication of the cast such as would be needed for x-rays or physical therapy treatments.*

Bone Mineral Content (BMC): *the amount of bone in a specified region, e.g. individual vertebra, femoral neck, etc.*

Bone Mineral Density (BMD): *1.) Bone mineral content divided by projected area (absorptiometry methods). 2.) Bone mineral content divided by volume element (computed tomography methods).*

Cast Syndrome: *superior mesenteric artery syndrome with disruption of circulation to the bowel. Occurs after application of a body cast and results in abdominal pain, diarrhea, and if unrecognized, severe problems.*

Compartment Syndrome: *circulation and function of tissue within a closed space are compromised by increased pressure within that space, with diminished oxygenated blood supply; may be due to over-exerted leg muscles, a tight bandage, or trauma-related injury. The syndrome may self-correct or progress, with eventual muscle necrosis (ischemia), loss of arterial blood supply, nerve palsy, or loss of limb. The most commonly affected compartments are the anterior leg (anterior compartment syndrome), volar forearm (leading to Volkmann ischemic contracture), and anterior thigh (rectus femorus syndrome).*

Constrictive Edema: *circulatory impairment causing disruption of normal venous drainage with resulting fluid accumulation in soft tissue and swelling distal to the point of constriction. Severe swelling may lead to neurovascular involvement and/or compartment syndrome.*

Contractures: *permanent shortening of soft tissue around a joint due to paralysis, spasm, or fibrosis; limits motion of the joint.*

Cortex: *the hard outer layer of bone.*

Decubitis Ulcer: *an area of breakdown of skin and/or subcutaneous tissue as a result of unrelieved pressure on a bony prominence or portion of the body resting on a firm surface for a long time. The lesions are as follows:*

Stage I: *only the dermis is involved.*

Stage II: *dermis and subcutaneous fat is involved.*

Stage III: *ulcer involves some deep fascia or muscle; bone not uncovered.*

Stage IV: *bone is exposed.*

Deoxyribonucleic Acid (DNA): *the strands in each cell's nucleus which contain the genetic information.*

Diarthrodial Joints: *joints which are lined with synovial tissue and in which bone is covered by hyaline cartilage. There is a thin layer of synovial fluid between the cartilage-covered surfaces of the two opposing bones. These joints allow free movement. An example would be the knee joint.*

Dropfoot: *when referring to a complication of cast treatment, applies to paralysis of the peroneal nerve resulting from pressure over the nerve causing inability to dorsiflex the ankle.*

Early Intervention: *therapy services provided for children from birth to age three. It usually includes physical therapy, occupational therapy, and speech therapy as needed by the individual child. The therapy may be given in an individual or a group setting and may be provided by an early intervention specialist, a specially trained nurse, an early education specialist, or by a licensed therapist.*

Fibrils: *the structure of a polypeptide, such as that forming collagen.*

Mosaicism: *when a person has different genetic information in various cell lines of the body. Example: skin cells do not test positive for OI but sperm or ovum do contain error in the gene for collagen, consistent with errors found in persons with OI.*

Muscle Atrophy: *loss of muscle tissue due to protracted disuse. It often occurs secondary to joint immobilization.*

Orthotic: *a device to straighten or support a part of the body, usually used in reference to the foot and/or ankle.*

Osteopenia: *any state in which bone mass is reduced below normal. This would include conditions of osteoporosis and osteomalcia.*

Osteosynthesis: *bone repair using internal fixation.*

Petrous Apex: *the portion of the temporal bone that holds the inner ear and ossicles.*

Pin Tract Infection: *direct bacterial contamination of area where pins have been used for external traction or skeletal fixation; could potentially lead to osteomyelitis.*

Polypeptides: *a protein made of amino acids.*

Positional Equino Varus: *mild clubfoot.*

Pressure Sores: *breakdown of skin and/or subcutaneous tissue that can occur because of direct pressure of displaced or bunched cotton padding under cast, creating pressure lasting usually in excess of four hours; often caused by patient inserting object in cast to reach an area that is itching from plaster dust in cast; decubitus ulcer.*

Subchondral: *pertaining to the area of bone just underneath the overlying layer of cartilage.*

Sudden Infant Death Syndrome (SIDS): *the diagnosis given when an apparently healthy infant dies from undetermined causes.*

Thrombophlebitis: *inflammation of a vein associated with thrombosis (blood clots) usually in the lower limbs. The clots can also become infected, i.e. septic thrombophlebitis.*

Tight Collimation: *the technique used during an x-ray examination in which the technologist selects the size of the area to be included in the x-ray in order to x-ray only the area of interest.*

Trabeculae: *the inner, spongy structure of bone.*

Univalve Cast: *cast split on one side to relieve pressure.*

NOTE: Some of the definitions of orthopaedic terms are adapted from <u>A Manual of Orthopaedic Terminology</u>, fifth edition, by C.T. Blauvelt and F.R.T. Nelson. Published by Mosby - Year Book, 1994.

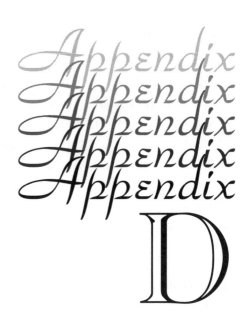

Concordance

E

F

G

◻ ◻ H ◻ ◻

◻ ◻ I ◻ ◻

⹂ ⹂ S ⹂ ⹂

⹂ ⹂ T ⹂ ⹂

U

V

W

X

Z

Appendix

Appendix
Appendix
Appendix
Appendix

E

Resources

The Osteogenesis Imperfecta Foundation, Inc. (OIF), is a non-profit organization which anyone can join for a modest membership fee. The OIF strives to support its members with information about day to day concerns of individuals with OI as well as to support research in the basic and clinical sciences related to this rare bone disease. There are many resources available through OIF, including a quarterly newsletter titled <u>Breakthrough</u>, pamphlets, videos, the book <u>Living With Osteogenesis Imperfecta: A Guidebook for Families</u>, personal contacts with families affected by OI, and of course, this book. Many areas of the United States also have active support groups affiliated with the OIF. During even numbered years, the OIF organizes a national conference on OI which is attended by hundreds of persons with OI and their families, as well as by medical professionals. The conference includes speakers and workshops on a variety of topics pertinent to OI. Contact the national office for membership, grant, or resource information.

> The Osteogenesis Imperfecta Foundation, Inc.
> 804 Diamond Avenue, Suite 210
> Gaithersburg, MD 20878
> 301-947-0083
> 800-981-2663
> fax: 301-947-0456
> E-mail: BoneLink@aol.com

Many topics relevant to persons with OI have yet to be fully explored. If you are interested in applying for research funds for either clinical or basic science projects, contact the national office listed above. The deadline for applications is November 30th each year.

OI Organizations Outside the United States

Australia

OI Association of Victoria   Phone number: 791-2059
    P. O. Box 34
    Vermont, 3133
    Victoria
    Australia

OI Society of New South Wales
    P.O. Box 401
    Epping
    New South Wales, 2121

OI Support Group of Tasmania
    Suzanne M. Cenin
    P.O. Box 97
    Brighton
    Tasmania, 7030
    Australia

Belgium

Zelfhupgroep OI, vzw
Meibloemstraat 12
B9900 Eeklo
Belgium

Phone number: 32-91-776727

Canada

Canadian Osteogenesis Imperfecta Society
128 Thornhill Crescent
Chatham, Ontario
Canada N7L 4M3

Phone number: 519-436-0025

Osteogenesis Imperfecta Canadian Society
c/o Beverly Treherne
807 Wasco Street
Coquitlam, BC
Canada V3J 5Z8

Denmark

Dansk Forening for OI (DFOI)
Gongesletten 23
DK 2950 Vedbaek
Denmark

Finland

Finnish OI Association
Pelimannintie 13
SF01390 Vantaa
Finland

The Finnish OI Society
Jouko Karanka
Rukokatu 21
SF33340 Tampere
Finland

France

Association de l'Osteogenese Imparfaite   Phone number: 33-35-923610
Secretariat du Registre
Hopital Nord
76570 SaintAustreberthe
France

Germany

German OI Society (GOIB)
OI Gesellschaft
Postfach 1546
63155 Mühlheim a.Main
Germany

Italy

Associazione Italiana Osteogenesi Imperfecta   Phone number: 049-650425
c/o Gadda Ersilio
Via Dietro Duomo 20
I 35139 Padova
20063
Italy

Japan

Network OI
c/o Susumo Kawamura
25-2 Fujimi-Cho
Itabashi, Tokyo 174
Japan

The Netherlands

OI Federation Europe (OIFE)   Phone number: 31-40-24-16-74
Luytelaer 1
Be Eindhoven
5632
The Netherlands

Vereniging Osteogenesis Imperfecta (VOI)
Postbus 389
4330 AJ Middelburg
The Netherlands

New Zealand

Brittle Bone Association of New Zealand, Inc   Phone number: 09-275-1872
c/o Richard Goulstone
69 Hall Avenue
Mangere, Auckland
New Zealand

Norway

Norsk Forening for OI (NFOI)
Postbox 114
Kjelsas
N 0411 Oslo
Norway

Peru

Asociacion Osteogenesis Imperfecta   Phone number: 4216234
Cervantes N 234103
Lima 33
Peru

Scotland

Brittle Bone Society   Phone number: 138-2204446
30 Guthrie Street
Dundee
DD1 5BS
Scotland

South Africa

South African Brittle Bone Association
37 Broadway
Westville 3630
Natal
South Africa

Sweden

OI Group of Sweden, RBU
Monika Kack
Hannebergsgatan 22
S-17147 Solna
Sweden

Switzerland

Schweizerische Vereinigung OI
c/o Frau Hanne Müller
Brandistrasse 25
CH 6048 Horw
Switzerland

Other Resources of Interest

Alliance of Genetic Support Groups
35 Wisconsin Circle Suite 440
Chevy Chase, MD 20815
800-336-GENE

American Academy of Orthopaedic Surgeons
6300 North River Road
Rosemont, IL 600184262
800-346-2267

American Council of Rural Special Education (ACRES)
University of Utah, Special Education Department
221 Milton Bennion Hall
Salt Lake City, UT 84112
801-585-5659

American Massage Therapy Association
820 Davis Street, Suite 100
Evanston, IL 60201-4444
847-864-0123

American Occupational Therapy Association (AOTA)
4720 Montgomery Lane
P. O. Box 31220
Bethesda, MD 20824-1220
301-652-2682

American Physical Therapy Association
1111 North Fairfax Street
Alexandria, VA 22314
703-684-2782

American School Health Association
7263 State Route 43
PO. Box 708
Kent, OH 44240
216-678-1601

American Society of Human Genetics
9650 Rockville Pike
Bethesda, MD 208143998
301-571-1825

Canadian Association for Community Living
Kinsmen National Institute York University
4700 Keele
Downsview, Ontario
Canada

Canine Companions for Independence
P.O. Box 446
Santa Rosa, CA 95402-0446
707-577-1700

Center on Education and Training for Employment
1900 Kenny Road
Columbus, OH 43210-1090
614-292-4353

Council for Exceptional Children
1920 Association Drive
Reston, VA 220911589
800-845-6232

Disability Resources, Inc.
Four Glatter Lane
Centereach, NY 117201032
516-585-0290

Dole Foundation for Employment of People With Disabilities
1819 H Street, NW   Suite 340
Washington, DC 20006
202-457-0318

ERIC Clearinghouse on Disabilities and Gifted Education
Council for Exceptional Children
1920 Association Drive
Reston, VA 20191-1589
703-620-3660

Exceptional Parent Magazine
209 Harvard St. #303
Brookline, MA 021465005
800-852-2884

Family Support Clearinghouse
2150 Hwy. 35, Suite 207 C
Sea Girt, NJ 08750
908-974-1144

Genetics Network of the Empire State
WCL&R, Room E299
P O Box 509
Albany, NY 122010509

Genome Action Coalition
317 Massachusetts Ave. NE #100
Washington, DC 20002
202-546-4732

Great Lakes Regional Genetics Group (GLaRGG)
328 Waisman Center
1500 Highland Avenue
Madison, WI 53705-2280
608-265-2907
(IN, IL, MI, MN, OH, AND WI)

Great Plains Genetics Service Network (GPGSN)
Delores Nesbitt
University of Iowa, Department of Pediatrics
200 Hawkins Drive
Iowa City, IA 52242
319-356-2674
(AR, IA, KS, MO, NB, ND, OK, SD)

Higher Education and Adult Training for People with Handicaps (HEATH)
HEATH Resource Center
One Dupont Circle N.W., Suite 800
Washington, DC 20036-1193
800-544-3284
202-939-9320

Job Accommodation Network
918 Chestnut Ridge Rd, Suite 1
P.O. Box 6080
Morgantown, WV 265066080
800-526-7234

Little People of America
P.O. Box 9897
Washington, DC 20016
888-572-2001

Mid-Atlantic Regional Human Genetics Network (MARHGN)
c/o Family Planning Council
260 S. Broad Street, Suite 1000
Philadelphia, PA 19102-3865
215-985-6759
(DE, DC, MD, NJ, PA, VA, WV)

National Academy of Orthopedic Nurses
E. Holly Ave. Box 56
Pitman, NJ 080710056
609-256-2310

National Association of Orthopaedic Technologists
3725 National Drive Suite 213
Raleigh, NC 27612
919-787-0755

National Association of Private Schools for Exceptional Children (NAPSEC)
1522 K Street N.W., Suite 1032
Washington, DC 20005
202-408-3338

National Center for Education in Maternal and Child Health Clearinghouse
2000 15th Street North, Suite 701
Arlington, VA 22201-2617
703-524-7802

National Center for Human Genome Research
9000 Rockville Pike Boulevard 38A605
Bethesda, MD 20892

National Center for Youth With Disabilities
University of Minnesota
Box 721, 420 Delaware St. SE
Minneapolis, MN 554550392
612-626-2825

National Easter Seal Society
230 West Monroe, Suite 1800
Chicago, IL 60606

National Information Center for Children and Youth With Disabilities (NICHCY)
P.O. Box 1492
Washington, DC 20013
800-695-0285

National Information Center On Deafness
Gallaudet University
800 Florida Ave NE
Washington, DC 20002

National Institute for the Disabled
National Rehabilitation Library
8455 Colesville Road Suite 935
Silver Springs, MD 20910

National Institute of Arthritis and Musculoskeletal and Skin Diseases (NIAMS)
National Institutes of Health
Dr. Joan A. McGowan
Natcher Building, Rm.5AS41
Bethesda, MD 20892
301-594-5005

National Institute on Disability and Rehabilitation Research (NIDRR)
Office address: 330 C Street SW, Washington, DC
Mailing address: 600 Independence Avenue, SW
Room 3060 MES
Washington, DC 20202-2572
202-205-9151
TTY: 202-205-9136

National Organization for Rare Disorders, Inc. (NORD)
P.O. Box 8923
New Fairfield, CT 06812
203-746-6518

National Osteoporosis Foundation
1150 17th Street, NW, Suite 500
Washington, DC 20036-4603
202-223-2226

National Parent to Parent
Marge Smith
P.O. Box 907
Blue Ridge, GA 30513
800-651-1151

National Rehabilitation Information Center (NARIC)
8455 Colesville Road
Silver Spring, MD 209103319
800-346-2742

ODPHP National Health Information Center
P O Box 1133
Washington, DC 20013
800-336-4997

Osteoporosis & Related Bone Diseases National Resource Center
1150 17th St., NW, Suite 500
Washington, DC 200364603
202-223-0344
800-624-BONE
Fax: 202-223-2237
TTY: 202-466-4315
Internet: http://www.osteo.org

Pacific Southwest Regional Genetics Network (PSRGN)
2151 Berkeley Way, Annex 4
Berkeley, CA 94704
510-540-2696
(CA, HI, NV)

Paget's Disease Foundation Inc.
200 Varick Street # 1004
New York, NY 10014
212-229-1582

Resources in Special Education (RISE)
9738 Lincoln Village Drive
Sacramento, CA 95827
916-228-2422

Rural Institute on Disabilities
52 Corbin Hall
The University of Montana
Missoula, MT 59812
800-732-0323
406-243-5467

Services for Independent Living, Inc.
25100 Euclid Ave., Suite 105
Braeburn Building
Euclid, OH 44117
216-731-1529

Shriner's Hospitals for Crippled Children
International Headquarters
2900 Rocky Point Drive
Tampa, FL 33607
Shriner's Hospital Referral Line
800-237-5055
800-282-9161 (in Florida)
Free orthopaedic treatment for many children under age 18.

Southeastern Regional Genetics Group (SERGG)
Emory University School of Medicine
2040 Ridgewood Drive
Atlanta, GA 30322
404-727-5731
(AL, FL, GA, KY, LA, MS, NC, SC, TN)

Special Education Resource Center
25 Industrial Park Road
Middletown, CT 064571520
860-632-1485

Special Kids
1080 North Delaware Avenue, Suite 702
Philadelphia, PA 19125
215-291-5560

Special Needs Resource Guide
P.O. Box 986
Sandy, OR 97055

Texas Genetics Network (TEXGENE)
Texas Department of Health
Bureau of Children's Health
1100 West 49th Street, Suite T 602
Austin, TX 78756-3199
512-458-7700

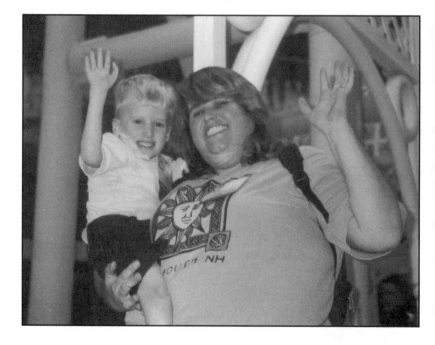

Another Important Resource Book

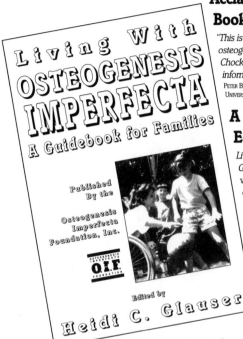

Acclaim for this Important Book

"This is the most thorough discussion of osteogenesis imperfecta ... ever written. Chock full of practical, accurate, and useful information ... long overdue."
PETER BYERS, M.D., DEPARTMENT OF PATHOLOGY AND MEDICINE, UNIVERSITY OF WASHINGTON, SEATTLE

A Word from the Editor

Living with Osteogenesis Imperfecta - A Guidebook for Families, offers people with osteogenesis imperfecta and their caregivers encouragement, comfort, knowledge, and a store of practical advice. Complete with an extensive resource guide listing, support organizations and resources. *Living with Osteogenesis Imperfecta - A Guidebook for Families,* is the book hundreds of people have been waiting for.